DR RUTH CILENTO

Anti-Cancer Cooking

Creative Feasts, Simply Delicious!

Hill of Content
Melbourne

This book is dedicated to the patients who are altering the course of their cancer through nutritional methods.

Read also: *Heal Cancer: Choose your own Survival Path*
by Dr Ruth Cilento, M.B.,B.S.,D.B.M.,D.Ac. FACNEM

Dr Ruth Cilento, M.B.,B.S.,D.B.M.,D.Ac. FACNEM
P.O. Box 129
Bracken Ridge, Queensland 4017

Cilento, Ruth, date.
Anti-cancer cookbook: creative feasts, simply delicious.

ISBN 085572 273 8

1. Cancer – Diet therapy – Recipes. 2. Cancer – Prevention.
3. Cancer – Nutritional aspects. i. Title.

641.5631

Acknowledgements
Illustrations, by permission from
The Health Revolution Cookbook by Ross Horne
The Colour Book of Cooking for One Edited by Valerie Creek
The Complete Cookbook: Colour Library Books

Contents

Preface

In 1982 my favourite cousin, my uncle and two dear friends died of cancer. I knew very little about cancer at that time and I felt frustrated, sad and helpless.

Always keen on research, I started reading everything I could in the literature that would give me clues on how this horrible disease begins and how to counteract it.

I was fortunate in having available the extensive library that my mother, Lady Phyllis Cilento, had collected in her lifelong practice of medicine, particularly in the fields of woman and child health, preventative medicine, and nutrition.

It soon became clearly evident that cancer is not just a series of lumps and ulcers, but a state of the whole body. It starts as a chemical imbalance and a change in cell membrane potential that causes cells to become stressed.

The chemical imbalance can be precipitated by many known factors, but also by many unknown changes that can occur insidiously while we appear to be healthy.

Of the 150 different identified types of tissue in the body about 120 contain cells with a nucleus or computer that tells the cell what work to do. Around each of these cells is a protective layer of ionised chemicals that keep the nucleus in a good state of health. Damage can occur when viruses, germs or chemical toxins broach this protective cell membrane.

It is a change in the working of the besieged nucleus that causes cancer. This change is made possible by deficiencies in the chemical protectors of the cell membrane. The chemicals of our body come almost entirely from our food and fluids. They are grouped into categories for identification and study purposes and include a vast array of substances.

Some of these are "essential", that is the body must take them in already made up into a form it can use. Others, although essential for health, can be manufactured by the body when needed out of its food or storage substances such as fat.

Food nutrients necessary for humans are:

Proteins

The ground substance of every cell, the building blocks of proteins are smaller molecules called amino acids — 22 in all, eight of which are **essential**.

Main sources of proteins and amino acids are in meat, liver, kidney and other animal parts, fish, eggs, milk and milk products and some in unrefined grains and legumes (the bean and pea family).

Among the diseases caused by protein lack the most evident is Kwashiakor, a lethal malnutrition of people in third world countries. Eighty per cent of those who die of this have concommitant cancer.

Carbohydrates

The unrefined grains and beans contain most starches and sugars in the best complete forms. When we refine them we change sometimes the combinations and upset the natural balance of substances there. For instance, carbohydrates always occur in combination with **fibre**, another essential of the body. When we refine a product such as sugar we take out the essential fibre and leave the "pure" carbohydrate that the body then may have difficulty using in the way we have evolved to use it. Imbalances here can cause diabetes, obesity and other metabolic diseases.

Fats

Fats are an essential part of every cell membrane in the body. There are many types of fats not all of them healthy. The body can convert excess carbohydrates to fat for storage. Our processed and refined modern diet provides too much fat in its worst forms and too much carbohydrate that is converted to bad forms of fat such as low density lipid (LDL) that can collect in the arteries as cholesterol plaques. However, the good fats with **essential fatty acids** such as linolenic (GLA), eicosapentaenoic acid (EPA) and docosahexaenoic acid (DHA) are the necessary protectors of all cell membrane integrity and are basic in preventing cancer, allergies etc. Some diseases of too much fat are obesity, hardening of the arteries and heart disease.

Fibre

The body uses fibre in many ways as we now know. It is not used just for the bulk that keeps the food in the bowel moving along. It also chelates out some toxic substances from the food and probably contains chemical constituents that act as catalysts in the digestive processes.

Fluid

An integral part of every cell for carrying of soluble or emulsified nutrients. We need a minimum of six to eight glasses of fluid a day. It may be in the form of pure water, but for those who have a limited appetite, pure freshly made fruit and vegetable juice is better. Herb teas also have a time-honoured gently therapeutic place.

Vitamins and minerals

The body cannot make vitamins and minerals but they are essential to its health and healing power. They are the catalysts that begin and end the thousands of chemical transactions that go on constantly in our bodies and in our brains. Without them we die. When they are deficient (as they are in the modern diet) we are "below par", not functioning to our best potential.

If we eat a full diet with no man-made chemicals in it we could gain all that we need. People with cancer find this very difficult. They are also depleted over years of polluted environment. Many need supplements which must be worked out individually by careful assessment.

Most anti-cancer nutritional programs have been created especially to provide the right nutrients in the most useful proportions and ratios.

The recipes collected in this book are some of those used by people with cancer who have been using tried and true programs of dietary change to bring the body back into chemical balance so that it can fight the cancer.

The process consists of:

1. Eliminating the toxic materials collected over years from our chemically polluted air, food and water.
2. Providing the fresh pure substances the body needs to build up the immune system with its defender cells and adrenal-pituitary axis for the control of stress.
3. Not providing substances in the diet on which cancer cells feed, e.g. sugar.
4. Restoring the depleted parcel of vitamins, minerals and other protective substances that counteract the spread of malignant cells.

Our good cells live by "oxidation". This is a process whereby the air we breathe and the food we eat provide the oxygen for energy and metabolism of each cell.

On the other hand cancer cells live by a fermentation process, they do not need oxygen and in fact use sugars and alcohols as the raw products for their growth.

That is one reason why we eliminate sugar and alcohol from our diets.

Raw fresh food provides most oxygen so 50-75 per cent of these diets are raw food. They also contain many cancer preventative substances.

For instance beta carotene is specifically needed for the living membranes of the respiratory system and other hollow organs. **Trace minerals** such as selenium and germanium are toxic in large amounts but healing in minute quantities and so on.

Although these are strong general guidelines, each person is different also, so that some people may be allergic to the very substances that could protect them most. Providentially nature has provided many sources for our necessary nutrients. Traditional food of different locations and cultures show us that people have worked out over centuries what was healthy for them to eat.

It is our altered tastes made by eating the commercially prepared, chemically polluted food full of empty calories "refined and processed junk" that has confused our natural selection of edible foodstuff.

Animals in their natural state will not eat poisonous weeds unless starving. Very young children given a varied choice of foods will choose a balanced diet if the food has not been artificially coloured, flavoured and preserved by chemicals. We are mostly unaware of the dangerous substances we are eating.

We cannot either rely on our sense of smell since (in most city dwellers) the olfactory sensitivity has been blunted by disease and pollution.

For those reasons it is necessary to **wash everything** you use to remove as much as possible any surface pollutants.

White flour, sugar, hard animal fats, alcohol, processed, refined and commerc- *ially processed foods containing artificial colouring, flavouring and preservatives such as cordials, pastries, cakes, jellies, salted, corned and smoked meats etc., should be eliminated from the diet altogether.*

Unsprayed produce grown with properly prepared compost is available in some areas — search for it. If possible grow your own. At least sprouts are easy to grow, inexpensive and do not take up much room.

Where possible collect your own rain water in buckets. Transfer to clean glass bottles or jars. Using water off the roof must be tempered by discretion. Find out whether there has been aerial spraying of crops with insecticides; constant hydrocarbons in the adjacent air from factories, diesel exhaust fumes, smoke, etc. Tank water will sometimes hold these, not to mention the droppings of resting pigeons.

Simple reverse osmosis water purifiers or activated carbon cartridge purifiers can be quite inexpensive. Do not use the chlorinating tablets recommended for killing germs in polluted water unless absolutely necessary. It is better to use prolonged boiling for sterilising water with bacterial or parasitic growth in it.

Your pure water should be reserved for making soup, herb tea or for reconstituting skim milk (if this is on your menu). Do not waste it for washing vegetables and fruit. These can be washed in ordinary water to which is added acetic acid (cheap white vinegar), one tablespoon to the pint or coarse salt, one heaped dessertspoon to the pint.

The types of recipes in this book correspond to the four main programs I used in my anti-cancer clinic: The Gerson Therapy; The Cilento Survival Plan; The Livingston Wheeler program and the Herbal therapy.

There is no easy description of these programs. After a careful assessment persons with cancer (and preferably helpers also) are taught to administer the treatment so they can persevere with this new way of life at home. Many have been

9

classed as "terminally ill" which means that they have been told by their doctor that surgery, radiation and chemotherapy will not cure their cancer.

Maximum nutritional aid plus minerals, vitamins and other food supplements can make the difference literally between life and death for these people, and can in most cases provide a better quality of life as well as further the time of survival in a happier state of mind.

In no way does anything in these programs fight with the treatment being given by the hospital doctor. In fact the nutritional impetus helps many of the other therapies to work better with less side effects.

Above all when preparing or sampling new food **expect to enjoy it**. The use of tempting garnishes and the blending of different **colours** all enhance the aroma and taste for someone with a feeble appetite. Make and serve only small portions to start. A little amount of food more often is better than a large amount that cannot be digested properly. Only juices between meals are best and are very easily absorbed.

A cheery atmosphere with happy faces and positive attitudes, no dissension and no distaste at meal-times should be the rule. Pleasant music or a comedy on television for those who are bedridden may be an answer.

These recipes are simply an adjunct to the programs and should in no way be construed as being a therapy in themselves or of any specific value without the rest of the knowledge necessary to fight the disease.

First were those I have used myself or in my mother's home. Others have been used with benefit in my Kelvin Grove clinic (now closed) for several years. In the past ten years many more patients with different tastes and ideas have added their recipes. I have tested most of them on myself and my family.

For specific guidelines in using the Cilento Survival Plan please read the first section of: "*Heal Cancer, Choose Your Own Survival Path*" by Dr. Ruth Cilento, (1993, published by Hill of Content, Melbourne). The day-by-day directions on pages 66 to 76 give particulars of meal construction.

Many of my patients who were considered to be terminally ill have been able to halt the spread of the disease. With Cancer I never say "cure". There is no such condition as "cure". Everyone of us has cancer cells in our body. It is the intricate job of our fantastic immune system to destroy these cancer cells, so keeping us in a state of equilibrium with our environment. It is **our** job to keep our internal and external environment free of pollution to withstand conditions that work against the immune systems. It is these conditions gradually breaking down our defences that cause the symptoms of our disease.

This book is about keeping the immune system strong and healthy by putting into the body, mind and spirit only the **positive** energies that food can provide. We have abundance all about us. Take it! Make it your own! Use it! It is there for YOU!

Acknowledgements

My thanks go to the many people who have shared their recipes with us and also to those who have tested, tasted and made helpful corrections.

For this edition special thanks go to Eileen Watson for providing, testing, writing out and distributing many of the recipes and to Pam Dew, Gwen Hussie, Denise Brien, May Broom, Annette Cloke, Peggy May, Paddy Webber, David Harker, Gwen Absalom, Lyn Brodie and to all those in the Quality of Life Group not to forget Rosemary Wetherell for typing and Helen Fowler and Marlene Lynn for overseeing arrangements.

Ruth Cilento, 1996

Some good food sources of vitamins and minerals

Vitamin A
Liver, egg yolk, fish oil.

Beta carotene
Dark green leafy vegetables, all yellow, orange and red fruits and vegetables.

Vitamin B1
Liver, brewer's yeast, all unrefined cereals, nuts and seeds, wheatgerm, legumes.

Vitamin B2
Liver, milk, brewer's yeast, eggs, kidney, cereals, nuts, mushrooms.

Vitamin B3
Liver, kidney, fish, brewer's yeast, eggs, wholegrains, legumes, nuts, mushrooms.

Vitamin B5
Liver, egg yolk, soybeans, some fish, brewer's yeast, cabbage family (such as broccoli), mushrooms, royal jelly, whole grains, nuts.

Vitamin B6
Liver, kidney, wheatgerm, seeds, fish, brewer's yeast, legumes, oatmeal, wholegrain, nuts.

Vitamin B12
Liver, kidney, oysters, fish roe, eggs.

Vitamin C
All fresh raw fruit and vegetable, especially citrus, strawberries, watermelon, cantaloupe, cabbage and fresh green leafy vegetables.

Vitamin D
Sunlight, fish liver oils, egg yolk, sprouts, milk.

Vitamin E
Wheatgerm, oils of nuts, cereals and seeds, fish roe, egg yolk.

Magnesium
Wheatgerm, nuts, legumes, whole grains, all dark green vegetables, dolomite, milk.

Potassium
All fresh fruits and vegetables, all legumes, oatmeal, potato, nuts, sweet potato, avocado, banana, apricot, mushrooms, molasses, fish, milk.

Calcium
Milk, yoghurt, cheese, dolomite, legumes, seeds, bonemeal, green leafy vegetables.

Sodium
Celery, kelp, salt, cheese, seafoods.

Sulphur
Garlic, onion, mushroom, cabbage family, celery.

Selenium
Liver, brewer's yeast, wheatgerm, egg, onion, garlic, kelp, goat's milk.

Zinc
Liver, oatmeal, legumes, fish, seeds and grains, leafy vegetables.

Iron
Liver, brewer's yeast, legumes, egg yolk, green leafy vegetables, wholegrains.

Copper
Liver, brewer's yeast, eggs, heart, prunes, almonds, legumes.

Essential fatty acids
Oils of seeds, grains and beans, especially cold pressed linseed (flax) oil, safflower, olive, corn.

Folic acid
Green leafy vegetables, liver, kidney, eggs, legumes, brewer's yeast.

Biotin
Brewer's yeast, sprouts, liver, kidney, milk, whole grain, rice, eggs.

P.A.B.A.
Brewer's yeast, whole grains, yoghurt,
liver, kidney.

Bioflavinoids
Pigment and pith of fruits and
vegetables, buckwheat, citrus.

Choline
Lecithin, brewer's yeast, liver, legumes,
whole grain, milk, eggs, brains.

Inositol
Lecithin, brewer's yeast, citrus, nuts,
whole grain.

B15 pangamic acid
Brewer's yeast, seeds, whole grain, liver,
kidney.

Nutrients needed for the Making of the Immune System

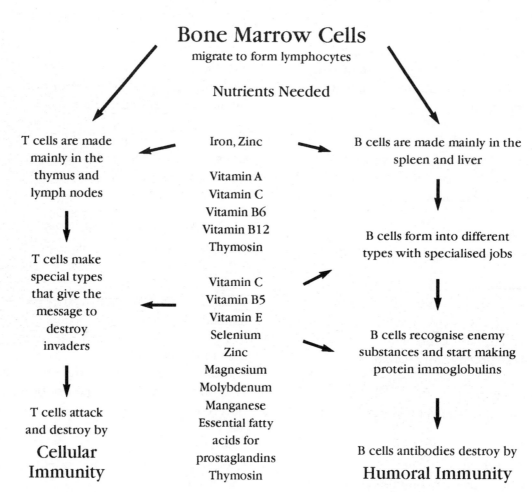

Bone Marrow Cells
migrate to form lymphocytes

Nutrients Needed

T cells are made mainly in the thymus and lymph nodes

Iron, Zinc

Vitamin A
Vitamin C
Vitamin B6
Vitamin B12
Thymosin

B cells are made mainly in the spleen and liver

T cells make special types that give the message to destroy invaders

Vitamin C
Vitamin B5
Vitamin E
Selenium
Zinc
Magnesium
Molybdenum
Manganese
Essential fatty acids for prostaglandins
Thymosin

B cells form into different types with specialised jobs

B cells recognise enemy substances and start making protein immoglobulins

T cells attack and destroy by

Cellular Immunity

B cells antibodies destroy by

Humoral Immunity

Something for Breakfast

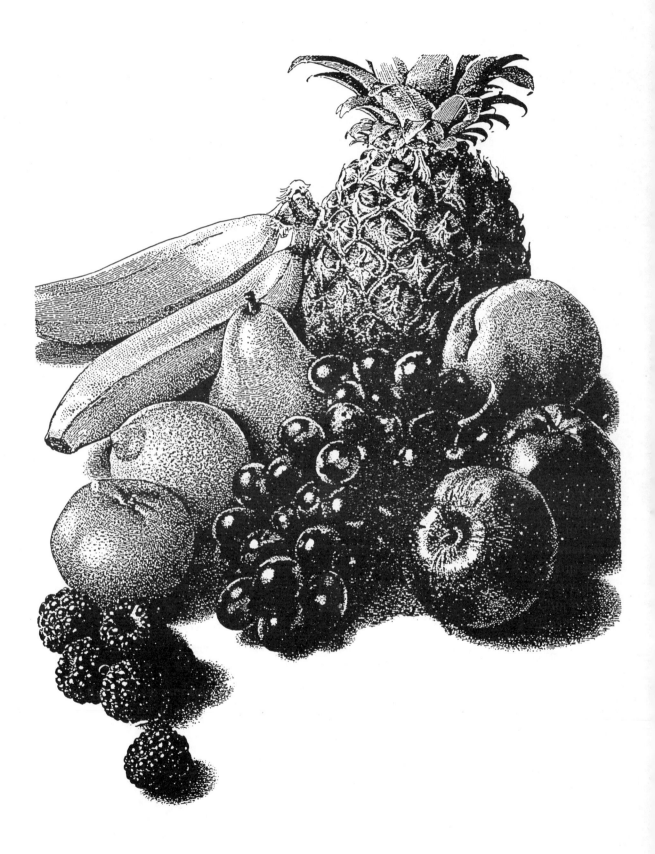

Liquid Breakfast Drink or Muesli or Mash

Serves 1 or 2

¼ cup Carnation skim milk powder plus 1-2 cups water or
   freshly prepared fruit juice
1 teaspoon, Brewer's yeast
1 teaspoon, Dolomite powder or 1 crushed tablet
2 teaspoons cold pressed Safflower Oil or cold pressed
   (flax) Linseed Oil
1 tablespoon Lecithin (as granules)
1 dessertspoon unprocessed bran
1 tablespoon wheatgerm
1-2 tablespoons natural yoghurt (recipe for making your
   own is found on p.106)
1 banana or other fresh fruit (fruit not necessary if made
   using fruit juice as the liquid)

Method: Place all ingredients into a blender goblet. Blend together thoroughly and drink immediately. As a muesli or mash add less fluid.

For people who are sensitive to bran this amount can be adjusted accordingly, for example, if constipated, increase it.

People with Candida (thrush) may find they are allergic to Brewer's yeast so this can be deleted.

Dried Fruit in Apple Juice

Dried fruit such as prunes, apples and apricots may be used
if no fresh fruit are available. Soak overnight, wash well and
then add fresh apple juice or other sweet fruit juice.

Method: Place fruit and juice in a saucepan, bring to the boil. Simmer till very tender. Pour into a bowl. Use hot or cold.

Flavours improve if left out for a day before eating. These may be added to the porridge when cooked or may be used as a puree by those with weak digestion after chemotherapy or surgery on the bowel.

Porridge with Prunes
in Apple Juice

Serves 2

¾ cup rolled oats (not quick oats) or any other flaked grains
   such as wheat, barley, rye, millet or rice. Oatmeal gives a
   smoother texture.
1½ cups skim milk or water
6 pitted prunes
½ cup apple juice

Method: Mix grain and liquid together. Leave to soak in the juice overnight. In the morning bring to the boil in a stainless steel saucepan, stirring constantly. Simmer for 10 minutes with the prunes before serving. By soaking the oats they do not require as much cooking and may be put through a sieve for people using a low fibre gruel diet.

Fruit Porridge

Serves 2

¾ cup rolled oats or other flaked grains
1½ cups pineapple juice or other juice such as apple,
   apricot, melon, etc.

Method: Mix oats and juice together. Leave to soak overnight. In the morning bring to the boil in a stainless steel saucepan, stirring constantly for 10 minutes.

   If preferred a mixture of half pineapple juice and half water can be used. With full strength juice it also makes an excellent dessert. Ideal served hot or cold.

   For those using the Gerson Diet the pineapple juice may be replaced with one of the other fruit juices suggested.

Muesli

2 cups rolled oats or other rolled grains such as rye, wheat,
    millet, barley, rice or a mixture of grains.
¼ cup unprocessed bran
1 cup wheatgerm
¼ cup lecithin granules
¼ cup chopped mixed dried fruits - raisins, sultanas,
    currants, prunes
¼ cup sunflower seeds
¼ cup sesame seeds

Method: Mix all ingredients together and store in an airtight container. Use for breakfast as required. ½ cup of the mixture makes a nice serving with either skim milk, fruit juice or water to moisten.

    For those allergic to wheat, delete wheatgerm, wheat bran or rolled wheat and use other grains. For people who are gluten sensitive, rice, corn, buckwheat (sorrel) or millet must only be used.

    Serve with fresh or stewed fruit, yoghurt and a teaspoon of honey.

Breakfast Fruit Cocktail

Serves 2

Select any fruits. Have a combination of colours and textures
    for interest and varied nutrition.
1 slice pineapple, chopped
1 slice pawpaw, chopped
1 kiwi fruit, sliced
1 orange, juiced

Method: Mix all ingredients together. Chill well before serving. Serve with a spoonful of banana yoghurt cream. For those using the Gerson Diet or having herbal mixture the pineapple and kiwi fruit may be replaced by melon and other available fruit.

Banana Yoghurt Cream

1 banana
¼ cup natural yoghurt

Method: Place both ingredients into a blender goblet. Blend to a smooth cream. Ideal served with the Breakfast Fruit Cocktail, fruit salads or any fresh fruit. Particularly nice with fresh strawberries. This may be made with frozen bananas.

Melon Cocktail

Watermelon
Rockmelon
Honeydew melon
Mint, chopped

Method: Chop up equal quantities of each type of melon available and mix together. Chill well before serving. Sprinkle with chopped mint just before serving or any other favourite herb. There is no contra-indication for using these melons together.

Lassi Drink (Nepal)

½ cup milk made with skim milk powder
½ cup reduced fat natural yoghurt
1 tablespoon or more of cold pressed flax or cold pressed
    safflower oil
2 teaspoons of honey
1 teaspoon natural vanilla essence
2 teaspoons rose water if liked

Method: Blend all together to make a "thick shake". This makes a delightful cold drink. Make double the quantity and keep half in refrigerator for next day. Do not heat it or the lactobacillus culture that makes the yoghurt will die. Bland non-acid fruit such as banana or pawpaw may be blended into it if liked.

Eggs

1 egg per person may be:

- Boiled with a soft yolk and served with wholegrain bread;
- Poached with a soft yolk. Served with wholegrain toast on a bed of spinach with cottage cheese on top;
- Added beaten to the liquid breakfast drink;
- Used in wheat cakes, (recipe given later)
- For those with a cholesterol problem it is best to have the egg yolk soft, others may have eggs in custard, quiche or scrambled.

Fish

60g fish per person – left-over cold baked fish from the previous day served with left-over vegetables, may be used for breakfast.

See also fish recipes.

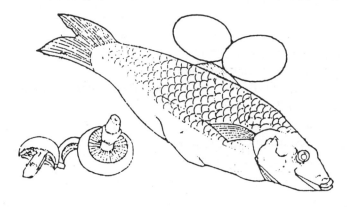

Cooking the Bean Family (legumes)

Dried Beans must be well cooked

Most fruits and vegetables can be eaten raw for their best nutritional value. But the legume family of vegetables should not be eaten raw or only partially cooked because of their toxic potential.

When dried legumes are thorougly cooked (soft inside, not crunchy), they contribute protein complex starches and B vitamins to the diet. If they are raw or under-cooked they can be dangerous for several reasons. Most raw legumes contain substances sometimes called "toxalbumins". When they are cooked, the heat of cooking changes the toxic chemicals into harmless substances, burns them up, or dilutes them in water.

Some of these substances are trypsin inhibitors, which prevent the enzyme trypsin from its proper action of protein breakdown. If trypsin inhibitors are ingested over a long period of time no matter how much protein you take in, it would be worthless to the body and normal growth could not take place. Raw soybeans and soy flour made from ground soybeans without heating contains these trypsin inhibitors. If you use soybeans they must be thoroughly cooked so that they can be mashed between your tongue and the roof of the mouth, otherwise they are not cooked enough. Use soy powder or soy flour which has been heat treated to remove these enzyme inhibitors.

Reasons for Cooking Legumes

Raw legumes, particularly soybeans, have a factor which can block the uptake of iodine by the thyroid. Some people recommend taking kelp as food or in tablets as a precaution if the diet is high in soybeans. Such seaweed products contain abundant iodine.

The anti-nutritional or toxic elements of legumes can be eliminated by appropriate methods of cooking, so that they have become wholesome dietary staples in many parts of the world.

Cooked legumes should not be the least bit crunchy. Do not think you are getting better nutrients from crisp, dried legumes as you are from crisp, succulent vegetables like zucchini or asparagus. Make sure your soybeans, chick-peas, and lima beans are **soft** inside.

Eliminating Flatulence

If you want to minimise digestive problems with the beans, you can discard the soaking water (and, if desired, the first cooking water). The basic cause of flatulence associated with beans in some people is their deficiency of some enzymes which break down into simple sugars the trisaccharide starches (raffinase and stachyose) normally found in beans.

The undigested trisaccharides provide food on the lower intestine for the natural bacterial flora which produce the carbon dioxide that causes flatulence.

Since the trisaccharides are water soluble, they may be removed from your bean dishes by discarding the soaking water after the beans have soaked at least three hours. There will only be a tiny loss of protein, minerals, and water soluble vitamins. You can go even further and discard the fresh water used to cook the beans for 30 minutes. Add new water and finish cooking.

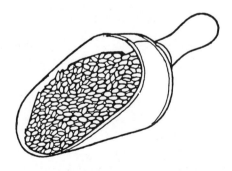

Cooking Hints

There are several methods of cooking beans.
Use the most convenient for you.

Soaking beans overnight

Soak washed and picked-over beans in a covered bowl in twice their volume of water. Refrigerate them in warm weather to prevent fermentation. (Split peas, lentils and blackeyed peas do not need soaking before cooking.)

To determine the number of hours ahead of serving time to start cooking the beans you have chosen, look at the chart and follow the instructions. Bring the beans in their pure water to the boil in a heavy saucepan, cover, lower heat, and simmer until tender (add more water to cover the beans if necessary). Remember that older beans that have been stored a long time are tougher and may take longer to cook than the specified times in the chart.

Short soaking beans

In a saucepan bring washed beans and $2\frac{1}{2}$ to 3 times their volume of water to a boil. Boil for 1 minute. Remove from heat, cover, and let stand for 1 hour. Then cook by simmering in a regular pot, covered as directed in the chart.

Quick no-soaking method

Wash a cup of dried beans and drop them with a spoon, just a few at a time, into a pot containing a quart of boiling water. Add only enough beans at a time so that the boiling does not stop.

This method allows the starch grains to burst, breaking the outside skins of the beans. The beans then cook quickly because they can absorb the hot water more rapidly. When all the beans have been put in the pot, cover, lower heat, and let the beans simmer until they are tender. (About the same time as that given in the chart overleaf).

Slow Cooker method

Beans soaked overnight or by the 1 hour method may be cooked in the slow cooker for 10 to 12 hours at low heat, or 5 or 6 hours at high heat. First pre-cook them for 1 hour by simmering on top of the stove.

Seasoning Beans

Only after the beans are cooked should you add tomatoes, molasses, or other seasonings. If you add any of these before cooking is finished, they can interfere with the cooking or toughen the beans.

21

Bean Cooking Timetable

The cooking times given are approximate. Beans vary in time needed for tenderising because of age or storage conditions. They get drier and tougher if stored long. Times given are for soaked beans (except for split peas, lentils, and blackeyed peas, which do not require soaking).

Type of bean	*Ordinary Cooking Pot*
Split Peas	30 minutes
Lentils	30 minutes
Blackeyed Peas	30 minutes
Speckled Peas	45 minutes
Small Limas	45 minutes
Whole Peas	1 to 1½ hours
Brown Peas	1 to 1½ hours
Large Lima Beans	1 to 1½ hours
Pinto Beans	2 hours
Kidney Beans	2 hours
Navy Beans	2 hours
Red Beans	2 hours
Black Beans	2 hours
Chickpeas	2 hours or more
Soybeans	2 hours or more

Bean Patties

Serves 2

1 cup cooked beans, soy or a mixture (useful to reserve
    some when making the bean soup or vegetable pies)
1 small onion, finely chopped
1 leaf silverbeet, finely chopped

Method: Mash beans, then stir through remaining ingredients. Form into four patties. Lightly brush over oven tray with safflower oil or use non-stick tray. Place patties on. Cook under a pre-heated grill until lightly coloured, then turn over and cook on second side.

As an evening meal these can be baked in the oven with vegetables to make a substantial meal. Soya beans should not be used by people on the Gerson program.

Wheat Cakes

Serves 2

⅓ cup Burghul (cracked wheat)
2 eggs, separated
¼ cup chopped parsley
2 shallots, finely chopped
2 large ripe tomatoes, cut into 4 slices each
Grated vegetables can also be used as a base for the egg
    yolk. Use the white to bind the vegetables together and
    follow the method given for the wheat cakes.

Method: Soak burghul in milk for 1 hour (for convenience it may be soaked overnight in the refrigerator so that it is ready to use in the morning).

Add egg whites, parsley and shallots, mix well.

Place sliced tomatoes onto an oven tray and then spoon the burghul mixture on these.

Cook under a pre-heated grill until lightly coloured, turn over and cook second side.

Make a depression in two of the cakes and place the egg yolks in. Return under grill just to warm through but do not harden.

Serve.

For those with gluten sensitivity corn meal (polenta) or cooked brown rice may be used instead of wheat.

Something for Lunch

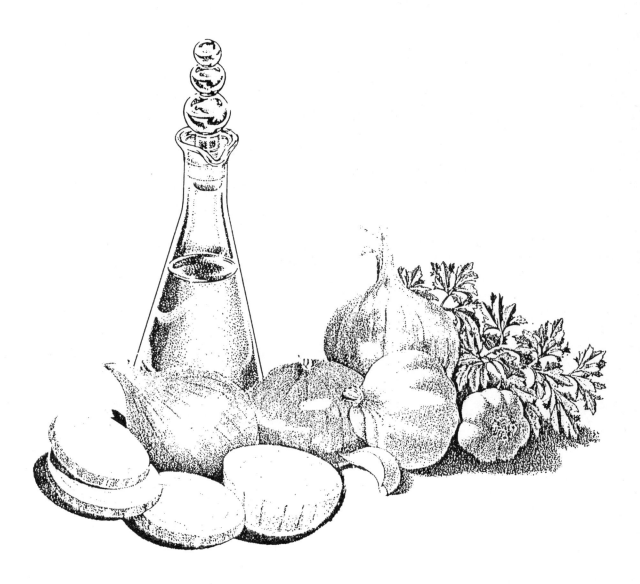

Hippocrates Soup

The basic Gerson direction is to use:

> 1–2 stalks celery
> 1 small leek
> 1 medium onion
> 2 tomatoes
> 2 potatoes

Method: Scrub vegetables well (do not peel), cut coarsely or grate. Cook slowly for three hours in enough water to cover.

We often begin with a tablespoon of lentils, barley or beans (e.g. red kidney or lima). Early in the day, add water and bring to the boil. Take off the heat and leave to stand, covered, for an hour. Alternatively soak them overnight.

Add the onion and your choice of herbs and bring to the boil, adding the stipulated vegetables while simmering. Any other vegetables may be used in addition to vary texture and colour — carrots, green beans, capsicum, pumpkin, sweet potato, turnip and broccoli are tasty. You may decide to add lemon juice before serving or press fresh garlic into the hot soup.

Keep any left-overs well covered in the refrigerator for no longer than 2 days.

Variations on Hippocrates Theme

Many different soups can be made by varying herbs, legumes and vegetables. For example, we make a delicious Pea and Pumpkin soup by starting with 1 tablespoon split peas (green and yellow), using rosemary, thyme and basil for herbs and adding lots and lots of butternut pumpkin (in addition to the Gerson vegetables). The pumpkin and peas both disintegrate to form a lovely thick base for the vegetables.

Mixed Bean Soup

2 cups mixed beans — select from kidney, blackeyed,
    haricot, lima, pinto, borlotti and chickpeas. (Not soy, they
    take much longer to cook than the others.)
2 cups tomato juice or 4 tomatoes processed in blender
2 large tomatoes, chopped
1 onion, sliced
2 carrots, diced
1 choko, diced
3 sticks celery, sliced
$\frac{1}{2}$ teaspoon ground coriander seeds
1 teaspoon ground cummin seeds

Method: Soak beans overnight in cold water (rain, purified or distilled water is best) or quick soak method. Cover beans with water and bring to the boil, then let them stand for 1 hour. Cook beans in water until tender. Pour off excess water. Add remaining ingredients, bring to boil and simmer for 25 minutes, or until the vegetables are cooked but still crisp. If more liquid is required add 1 cup of water.

This soup has a beautiful flavour and is nice with lots of whole beans and chopped vegetables in a tasty thin liquid. If preferred split peas can be included in the bean mix and on cooking these will soften and thicken the soup. This soup can be frozen in serving size portions if desired. For people on the Hoxsey, Herbal or Kelley programs delete tomatoes and juice. Use vegetable water or vegetable stock (recipe given later) and 2 capsicums diced.

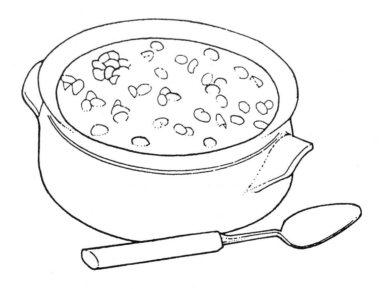

27

Vegetable Juice Soup

Prepare the following juices using a standard juice extractor.

1 cup pumpkin juice or diced pumpkin
1 cup carrot juice
1 cup potato juice or diced potato
1 cup apple juice
1 cup tomato juice
$\frac{1}{4}$ cup celery juice
$\frac{1}{2}$ cup pearl barley
$\frac{1}{2}$ cup chopped onion

Method: Pour juices into a saucepan with diced pumpkin, potato, $\frac{1}{2}$ cup pearl barley, 2 cups water and $\frac{1}{2}$ cup chopped onion, simmer and keep stirring until it thickens. Flavour with lemon juice and/or garlic and fresh basil.

Pumpkin Soup

3 cups diced pumpkin
2 cups diced sweet potato
$\frac{1}{2}$ cup chopped onion
$\frac{1}{4}$ cup pearl barley or $\frac{1}{2}$ cup cooked rice
$\frac{1}{4}$ teaspoon freshly grated ginger

Method: Mix all ingredients with 6 to 8 cups of water and simmer until rice is cooked. Fresh basil can be added before serving.

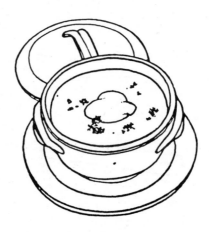

Cream of Vegetable Soup

1 onion, finely sliced
1 carrot, coarsely grated
1 potato, coarsely grated
1 sweet potato, coarsely grated
2 sticks celery, sliced
1 capsicum, sliced
2 zucchinis, coarsely grated
¾ litre vegetable stock (recipe given later)
2 tablespoons rice flour
¼ cup chopped parsley
2 tablespoons of water, rain, purified or distilled

Method: Place sliced onions into a large saucepan with 2 tablespoons of water. Cover and gently cook until tender. Add remaining vegetables and stock. Bring to the boil and simmer for 20 minutes or until vegetables are just tender. Mix rice flour with a little water to form a thin paste. Stir into the soup and boil for 5 minutes stirring constantly. Add parsley just before serving.

Note: Select small vegetables or increase the amount of stock and thicken. Make to suit individual taste, but there is a large concentration of vegetables in a very flavourful liquid using the above quantities. It is also nice served without the thickener and the parsley as a light soup. The soup can also be thickened with arrowroot, which gives a clear thick soup.

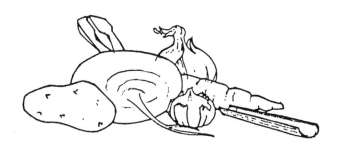

Tomato and Rosemary Soup

4 large tomatoes
1 large potato
2 pinches rosemary (preferably fresh)
Small amount of water

Method: Cook all ingredients in a stainless steel saucepan with lid on over low heat. When potato is soft, soup is cooked. Blend.

Lentil Soup

$2\frac{1}{2}$ cups red lentils
$2\frac{1}{2}$ cups vegetable stock
1 onion, chopped
2 cloves garlic, crushed
2 large tomatoes, skinned and chopped
1 bay leaf
$\frac{1}{2}$ teaspoon oregano
1 teaspoon lemon juice

Method: Soak lentils in cold water overnight. Rinse. Put into saucepan and pour in stock. Add onion, garlic, tomatoes, bay leaf and oregano. Bring to the boil, cover and simmer for 35 minutes. Add vinegar or lemon juice. Garnish with parsley and lemon.

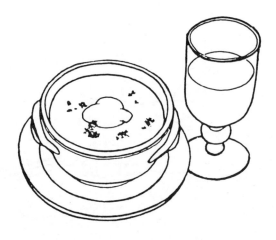

Vegetable Lunch

1 avocado
2 oranges, 1 segmented and 1 juiced
1 small carrot or beetroot, grated
1 stick celery, finely chopped
2 wholegrain muffins or unleavened breads

Method: Mash avocado to a smooth consistency. Stir in orange juice. Mix through remaining ingredients.

Split muffins in half and divide avocado between them.

Serve straight away. This also makes a good dip.

Fish in Vegetable Sauce

1 onion
1 carrot
2 tomatoes
1 red capsicum
Fresh mixed herbs — oregano, parsley and thyme are a nice
  mixture
2 fresh mullet fillets — tailor or tuna are also ideal

Method: Place first five ingredients into a food processor and process to a fine consistency.

Pour into a pan. Cover and cook gently for 20 minutes or until soft. No oil is necessary, there is sufficient moisture to prevent sticking.

Wash and carefully remove any scales or bones from the fish. Place it on top and continue cooking for a further 10 to 15 minutes, until the fish looks opaque and just starts to flake. Timing obviously depends on the thickness of the fish.

Note: If the sauce cooks too quickly and becomes too thick add a little water to correct. Any fish used should be fresh, never frozen, tinned, preserved or smoked.

Egg Noodles

(see also pasta dishes)

1$\frac{1}{2}$ cups wholemeal flour
2 eggs, beaten
2 to 3 tablespoons water

Method: Place flour into a bowl, add the eggs and 1 tablespoon of water. Mix to a firm dough, adding more water if necessary. Knead until smooth. Divide into three pieces and roll out as thinly as possible. Cut into $\frac{1}{2}$ cm strips and hang up to dry, whilst preparing next step.

Place 4 cups water in a saucepan and bring to the boil. Add the noodles and cook for 1 minute only. Drain well, al-dente.

To Serve — Toss in a little curd cheese, pour on some tomato sauce (see sauces) and sprinkle with chopped basil.

Redolent Reef Fish

Serves 2

200g fresh white fish, coral trout, sweetlip, etc.
1 onion, sliced
2 lemons or 4 times juiced, or a combination
3 sprigs dill, chopped
1 clove garlic, crushed
Grated raw ginger if liked

Method: Remove skin and cut fish into thin slices. Place fish and remaining ingredients into a glass oven dish, cover. Bake in a moderate oven $\frac{1}{2}$ to 1 hour. The fish is ready as soon as it looks opaque. Just before serving slices of fresh avocado, tomato or capsicum may be added. Any fish used should be fresh, never frozen, tinned, preserved or smoked.

Tasty Protein Pie

Serves 6

1 quantity of Tofu and pumpkin pastry
* 1 small carrot or beetroot, grated
1 small onion, finely sliced
1 leaf silverbeet, finely sliced
1 small sweet potato, grated
1 stick celery finely sliced
1 cup <u>cooked</u> soy beans or other cooked beans such as lima,
    haricot, kidney, pinto, borlotti, blackeyed or chickpeas.
½ cup cooked brown rice
Nutmeg to taste
*The beetroot gives a much nicer flavour to the pie but it
    does make the filling quite red in appearance.

Method: Roll out half pastry to baseline on a 22cm pie dish. Mix remaining ingredients together with grated nutmeg to taste. Don't overdo the seasoning, nutmeg can be a little over-powering in flavour.

Pile filling on top of pastry base, roll out second half of pastry and use to cover pie. Seal edges with a little water. Bake at 180°C (350°F) for 45 minutes. Ideal served hot, warm or cold.

Note: Individual size pies are excellent for picnics. This quantity of filling will fill approximately 9 to 10 individual pies. To have sufficient pastry make 1 ½ times the quantity of Tofu and Pumpkin pastry. Tofu pastry remains the crispest of all the pastries even when cold.

If there is some filling mixture left over, this is very nice stir-cooked in a pan with 1 tablespoon of water on a medium heat. Stir, then cover and leave to cook until warmed through and vegetables are softened.

Tofu pastry and soybeans should not be used by people on the Gerson program. Substitute any other beans suggested above and see recipes for pastry given later where cottage cheese is used as a substitute for Tofu.

Baked Fish in Cottage Cheese

Fillets of fish
Cottage cheese
Basil or other herbs
Crushed raw macadamia nuts

Method: In a baking dish place a fresh de-boned fish, cover with cottage cheese.
Sprinkle with basil or other herbs and generously top with macadamia nuts.
Bake in a moderate oven until cooked.

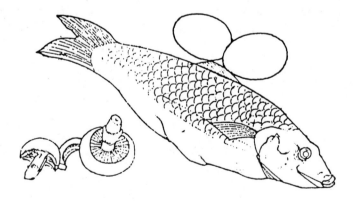

Paella

Serves 8-10

Combining rice and vegetables with grain and legumes.

2 large onions, peeled and roughly chopped

3 large capsicums (sweet peppers), the inner membranes
 and seeds removed and cut into strips

5 large cloves garlic pressed

1 lb (455g) fresh tomatoes, chopped

8 oz (225g) green beans

20 chopped raw almonds

1 tablespoon tomato puree

1 teaspoon paprika (not hot)

2 oz (55g) mushrooms

A few strands of saffron or $\frac{1}{2}$ teaspoon powdered saffron
 (optional)

1 lb (455g) brown rice

2 pints stock (see recipe)

4 oz (110g) fresh peas

1 lemon

Method: Soak the saffron in some of the stock for about 20 minutes. Use a large thick based pan, add a little pure water to the chopped onion and cook gently until they are soft. Then add the strips of peppers, the garlic and paprika. Cook gently for another couple of minutes, then add the tomatoes, with the tomato puree, mushrooms and rice. Stir to mix all the ingredients, then add the stock, cover the pan tightly and simmer very gently for about 35-40 minutes, until the rice is cooked. Meanwhile, top and tail the beans and cook them and the peas lightly. When the rice is ready, stir in the beans, the peas and the lemon rind and juice to taste. Decorate with chopped raw almonds.

Serve on its own, with a salad or decorated with grated carrot, parsley and watercress.

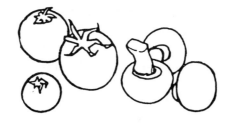

Seafood with Salad

Serves 2

200g fresh thick fish fillet, cut into thin strips or cubes
1 teaspoon apple cider vinegar or lemon juice
1 teaspoon chopped fresh parsley
Salad — prepare a large mixed green salad of your choice.
    Use a selection of salad leaves such as endive, nasturtium,
    watercress, mignonette, spinach, broccoli flowers with oil
    and vinegar dressing.

Method: Place fish in a bowl and sprinkle on vinegar or lemon juice and herbs. Toss well. Grill fish in a heat proof dish. As the slices are thin this is very quick. Pour dressing on salad and toss. Divide onto two plates. Place cooked fish on top and serve.

For people with allergies to yeast use lemon juice instead of vinegar. Any fish should be fresh, never frozen, tinned, preserved or smoked.

Stuffed Tomato

1 firm tomato per person
Stuffing for 4 serves
½ cup cooked brown rice or buckwheat
½ small onion, finely diced (optional)
½ cup chopped silverbeet or lettuce
½ cup diced broccoli
Chopped fresh herbs
Linseed oil and caraway seeds

Method: Slice top off tomatoes, scoop out insides, heat chopped onion in a dry saucepan until soft, mix in all ingredients including a few tablespoons of juice from the tomato. Pack this mixture into the hollow tomatoes, place in an open casserole dish containing a cup of water, and bake at 375°C until tomato flesh is soft. Eat hot or cold.

If your diet permits, top with ground almonds and or cottage cheese and chopped parsley.

Steamed Vegetables and Rice

1 cup brown rice is boiled in 2½ cups of water until steam holes appear in the rice. Cover and simmer on low heat until rice is soft and fluffy. Choose from a good selection of vegetables to obtain a colourful variety, e.g. broccoli, carrot, parsnip, corn, green beans.

Chop all vegetables into bite sized pieces, 1 to 2 cups per person is sufficient. Steam or cook in a minimum of water until soft enough to eat (or to suit your digestion). Combine vegetables and rice.

For flavouring experiment with any of the following:

> Lemon juice, tomato juice, crushed garlic, caraway seeds,
> basil, mixed herbs, oregano, a small amount of fresh grated
> ginger, thinly chopped shallots or chopped parsley.

They will all give a distinctive flavour. Add cold pressed flax or olive oil after cooking this dish, for a nutty flavour.

Zaje (Saya) Soup

1 bunch spinach washed and chopped
1 large potato nicked and chopped
Fennel tops and a pinch of cummin seeds
1 cup Italian broad beans
Little pinch of bicarb of soda

Method: Soak beans overnight in bicarb and water. Rinse thoroughly and discard water. Cook all ingredients in together in a stainless steel pot at low heat until potato and beans have "mushed in".

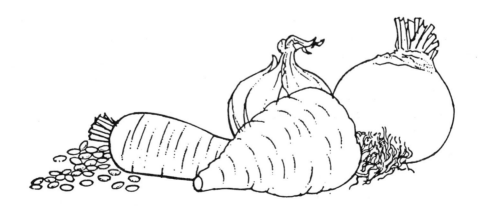

Potatoes and other Staples

Mashed potato is a nourishing dish on its own or may be used as a topping on vegetable, fish, turkey, rabbit, liver or kidney casseroles or it may be used to thicken soups or sauces.

Different staple starches are used in various parts of the world and such is the resilience of the human body that people may maintain good health and resistance to disease with the variety of widely differing foods available. Some of the staples foods are; wheat, corn, rice, oats, beans, yams, potatoes, cassava, bananas, peanuts and sago. Most staples need the adjunct of other vegetables, oils, fruits and the protein foods to provide the full nutritional requirements. In Australia we have an abundance of foods that give us multiple choices to give perfect health.

Potato Pastry

1 egg beaten
1½ cups mashed potato
1½ cups wholemeal flour
½ cup skim milk (mixed Carnation skim powder)

Method: Combine beaten egg and potato. Add flour and milk. Let stand ½ hour before rolling.

Quiche

4 eggs
1 cup Carnation milk
½ cup wholemeal plain flour
Onion chopped finely
Spinach and capsicum (sweet pepper) chopped
Asparagus cut up
Cottage cheese

Method: Blend the first 3 ingredients together until smooth. Arrange the next three in a greased oven dish. Pour over blended mixture. Top with cottage cheese. Bake in a moderate oven for 20 minutes or until set. Serve with toast and salad.

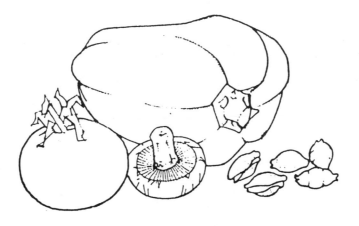

Tasty Lentil Lunch

1 cup dry lentils (soak lentils for 2 hours in pure water, bring
    to the boil and simmer till tender. Meanwhile mix together
    the first six of the following:)
1 tablespoon of mint
1 tablespoon of parsley
1 teaspoon of grated onion
1 tablespoon of cottage cheese
1 teaspoon of fenugreek
6 cardamon seeds
4 tablespoons of yoghurt

Method: Stir over low heat in non-stick frypan till brown. Add yoghurt (do not
cook yoghurt). Fold into the lentils and serve garnished with chives.

Aunt Ruby's Sweet Potato Soup

3 medium to large sweet potatoes (salmon coloured ones are best)
2 cloves of garlic, chopped finely
1 teaspoon curry powder
1 dessertspoon of arrowroot
Pure water

Method: Into a large stainless steel saucepan put the sweet potato, peeled and
diced into chunks, the garlic and curry powder. Cover with filtered or purified
water into which the arrowroot has been stirred. Stir until boiling strongly, then
turn heat down and simmer till tender. Mash, or puree in a blender, add made up
skim milk, yoghurt or cream, if too thick, and garnish with chives.

Classical Cabbage Rolls

Serves 4 with wheat or rice

8 large cabbage leaves or bok choy or grape leaves
4 oz (110g) burghul wheat or brown rice
½ pt (0.3 lt) stock (see recipe)
1 onion, peeled and finely chopped
1 clove garlic, chopped and pressed
4 tablespoons cottage cheese
2 tablespoons washed sultanas
½ teaspoon ground cummin
1 teaspoon chopped oregano or mixed herbs

Method: Blanch the cabbage leaves for 7 minutes in boiling water. Drain and separate. Pour the stock over the wheat or rice and leave for ½ hour to soak. Meanwhile, put a little pure water in a pan, add the onion and cook until just soft. Mix in the other ingredients and stir 1 minute over a gentle heat. Spread out each cabbage leaf, put 2 or more teaspoons or mixture per leaf. Wrap the leaves up into neat parcels. Place them with their tucked-over edges down, to keep the parcels intact. Either steam them for ½ hour or cook them over a gentle heat in a little water, with the pan covered for the first 20 minutes, then uncovered to allow the liquid to evaporate.

Serve with home made tomato sauce (see recipe).

Vegetables Sauces *(See also Sauces)*

Steamed vegetables have a delicious flavour if cooked carefully by themselves. However for variety various sauces can be made by putting vegetables, fresh or cooked into the blender and using the puree as a sauce.

Simply mix in some fresh herbs and when your diet allows it some butter mixture can be used.

This tomato with basil is delicious!

Blend tomato and fresh basil, chop up one tomato and puree in a blender or food processor with a sprinkle of basil, heat up to desired temperature for eating and pour over vegetables.

The liquid from a thin soup can be spooned over vegetables to impart a new flavour.

Gluten Free Soups

Bases for soups can be made from potato, pumpkin, rice, corn, root vegetables, and legumes (peas and beans).

Soak and cook beans as described previously. (See cooking the bean family). Add one diced onion and 4 diced tomatoes for each 2 cups of cooked beans. Simmer for 1 hour. Rice, corn and millet as liked may be added at the same time as the tomatoes. Mix in some sweet basil just before serving, any broth left over will provide a sustaining drink. Any vegetables can be added to this dish, either add them at the same time as the tomatoes, or steam them lightly and serve with the beans.

Lentils with Cabbage, Bok Choy and Potato

Soak lentils for 2 hours in water. Discard water. For each 2 cups of dried lentils add 2 medium potatoes diced, 1 big leaf of cabbage or bok choy chopped and 1 chopped onion. Bring to the boil and then simmer until the lentils are soft.

Serve hot with a squeeze of lemon juice.

Lentil Pie

1 cup dry lentils
Tomato juice to cover
1 onion, chopped
3 diced tomatoes
Herbs of your choice (sage, rosemary and dill are tasty)
Crushed garlic (optional)
Rolled oats pastry
Sliced tomatoes for garnish

Method: Cook lentils, juice, onion, tomatoes and herbs until lentils are soft and mixture fairly dry. Fill pie dish with cooked mixture, top with pastry, sprinkle with crushed garlic if you wish, garnish with sliced tomatoes and cook in hot oven till pastry is golden brown. Serve with salad, hot or cold.

Something for Dinner

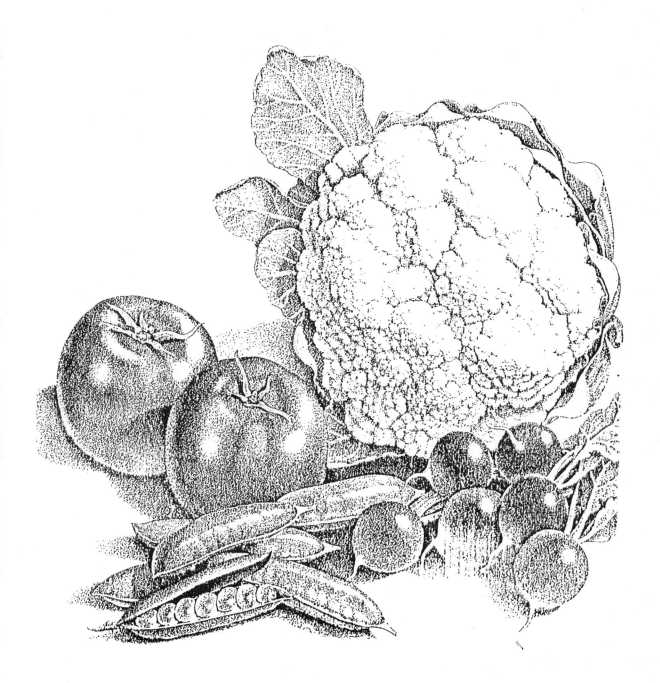

Cooking Turkey

Turkeys are sensible birds, they refuse to grow in batteries and insist on being free range. They are not as disease prone as chickens and much fussier in their eating habits. Because their flesh contains very little fat, they do not collect so much pollution from the environment, but the meat does tend to dry out in cooking, so it is best to use recipes that seal in the flavours and juices.

Left over meat may be frozen and can be used in any way mince meat is used.

Roast Turkey

It is possible to buy parts of the free range bird in many places if the whole turkey is too big. Stuffing with breadcrumbs, onion, herbs, prunes, seasoning and egg binder is usual.

Brushing the outside of the roast with seasoning and orange juice before wrapping it in foil will hold in delcious flavours. Cook for first half hour or so in a fast oven, then turn the heat lower and continue until when the thickest piece of roast is tested with a skewer there are no pink juices. About 2 hours at 450°F or 3 hours at 325°F for each 6 lbs if the oven is hot when you put the roast in.

Serve with sauces or bread, parsnips, greens, fruits such as apple, orange or berries or vegetable purees cooked or raw. Bake other vegetable dishes in the oven at the same time.

Left-overs can be used in fricassees, casseroles, minced in patties or as cold cuts of roast in salads or sandwiches.

Rabbit may be roasted or baked in the same way as turkey.

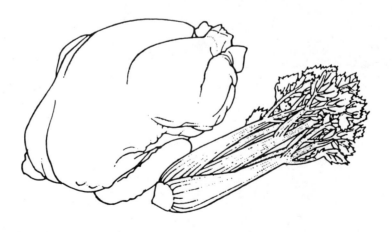

Rabbit Stew

1½ lbs (680g) rabbit cut into pieces

2 large onions peeled and chopped

8 oz (225g) brown rice, washed and soaked for at least an
   hour

2¼ pints (1 litre) pure water or stock

Corn kernels cut off 2 cobs

3 sticks of celery, chopped

3 large potatoes, quartered

3 large tomatoes chopped

1 teaspoon mixed herbs or 2 teaspoons of chopped fresh
   herbs such as marjoram and thyme

Method: Put a little water with the rabbit pieces and onion in large coated pan on medium heat. Stir and turn to prevent burning until cooked evenly. Add the stock, rice, rest of the vegetables and herbs. Simmer for 1½ hours or until the meat is leaving the bone. Thicken with arrowroot or mashed potato if there is too much liquid, add more stock if it is too dry.

Serve with salad, bread or dry baked potatoes. Cooked beans may be used instead of rice.

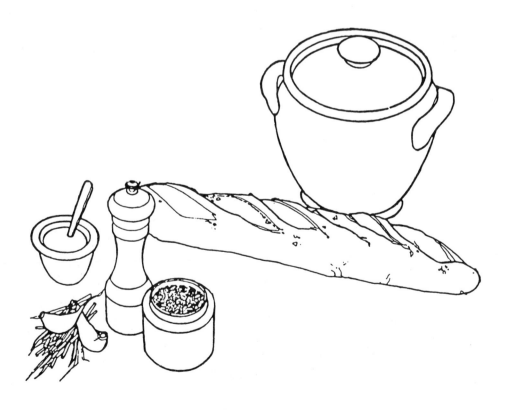

Fish in Pumpkin Sauce

Serves 2

1 small onion, sliced
¼ cup water
1 cup pumpkin, roughly chopped
3 tomatoes
1 capsicum (red or green pepper)
2 white fish fillets (fresh, washed, scaled and de-boned)

Method: Place onion in a pan with 1 tablespoon of water. Cover and cook gently until soft.

In a food processor place pumpkin, tomatoes and half the capsicum. Process to a fine consistency. Pour into pan and simmer, covered, for 10 minutes. Slice remaining capsicum. Add fish and sliced capsicum to pan adjusting consistency of sauce with remaining water if necessary.

Cook covered for a further 10 to 15 minutes or until the fish turns opaque and just starts to flake.

Serve with small potatoes boiled whole and a large fresh mixed salad.

For people on the Herbal or Kelley program, delete the tomatoes and substitute another capsicum.

Any fish used should be fresh, never frozen, tinned, preserved or smoked.

Kidneys with Apple Gravy

Serves 2

6 kidneys, lamb
1 apple, sliced thinly
3 sprigs mint

Method: Remove fat and membranes from kidneys. Split in half but don't cut all the way through. Place a piece of apple and some mint leaves onto each kidney. Place remaining apple slices in an oven bag or a casserole dish with a tight fitting lid. Arrange kidneys on top of apple slices and secure bag with metal tie. Puncture bag twice near the tie.

Place an ovenproof dish and bake for 40 to 45 minutes at 160°C (325°F). When cooked remove the kidneys and pour contents of bag into a blender to make the sauce. Pour sauce over kidneys and serve.

As a variation, an onion can be used in place of the apple or it can be added as well.

Liver with Ginger Yoghurt Sauce

Serves 2

1 orange, juiced
1 teaspoon grated green ginger
200g lambs liver, sliced thinly
3 stalks celery, sliced
10 button mushrooms, sliced or 1 sliced onion
2 tablespoons natural yoghurt

Method: Pour orange juice and green ginger into frypan. Heat on a medium setting. Add liver and cook until just cooked through. **Do not overcook** or it will become grainy and tough.

Remove the liver. Add all the vegetables and stir through juices, cook covered for about 5 minutes or until vegetables are just tender. Remove pan from heat. Stir in yoghurt gently.

Serve with boiled brown rice. Delete the mushrooms and add 1 sliced onion instead if on the Gerson program.

Liver and Onion

1 lamb's liver, young and fresh
1 large onion, chopped finely
3 tablespoons fresh chopped parsley
1 tablespoon wholemeal flour seasoned with herbs to taste
1 large tomato, chopped
Oregano leaves, fresh or dried
Water

Method: Put 3 tablespoons of water into a wok or stainless steel pan. Simmer the onion, herbs and tomato in it until onion starts to soften. Slice liver thinly. Dredge with seasoned four. Cook gently on top of vegetables, turning often until colour changes. Add oregano, stir in and simmer briefly. Add more water if it is too thick.

Serve covered with parsley.

Lamb's Liver Paté

1 lamb's liver
1 cup buttermilk
1 teaspoon dried or finely chopped fresh mixed herbs
1 teaspoon Bernard Jensen's vegetable seasoning powder
2 eggs
1 clove garlic, crushed

Method: Peel liver. Cut into slices. Dredge both sides of each slice with seasoning powder. With a little water in pan, sear quickly in a wok or coated pan. Watch it change colour, then cool. Mince the liver. Beat in the buttermilk, eggs, garlic and herbs. Fill a small deep casserole dish with mixture, cover top with lid or foil, stand in a pan of hot water. Cook one hour in moderate oven. Remove and press with heavy weight until quite cold. Turn out whole or serve in a crock. Spread on a wholemeal toast. Keep well refrigerated. Lasts no more than 3 days.

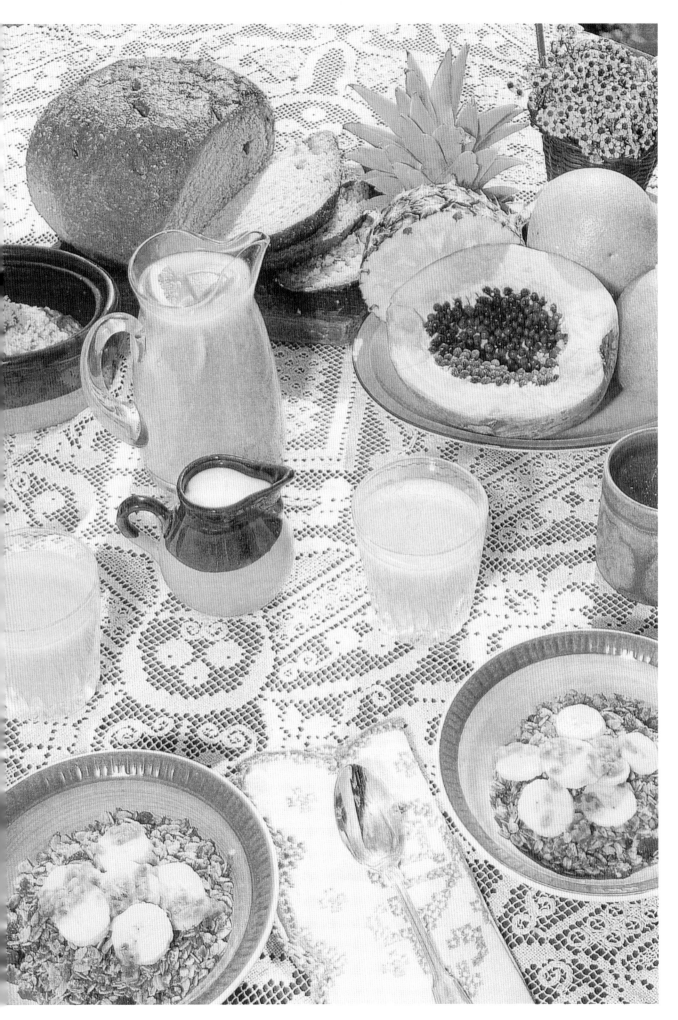

Muesli and breaskfast foods

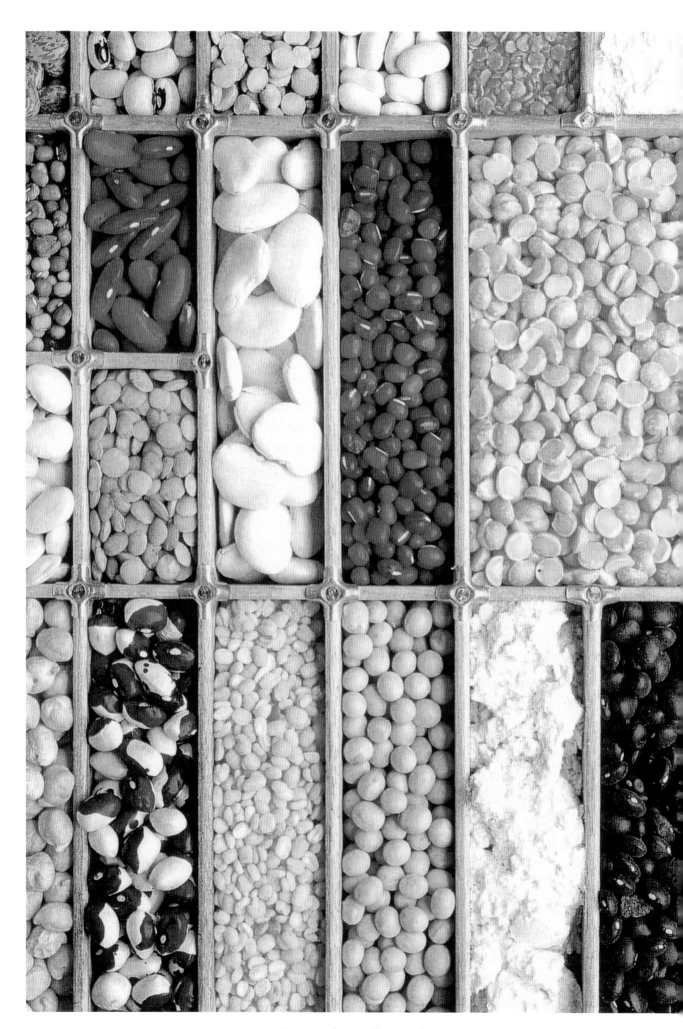

Beans and peas (legumes)

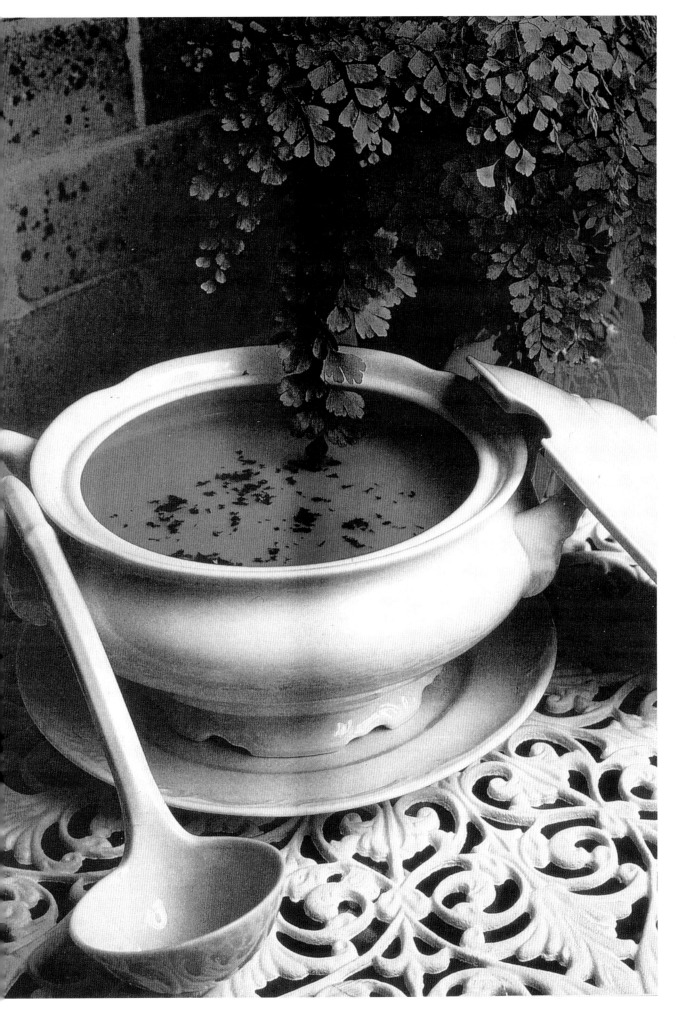

Tomato and rosemary soup

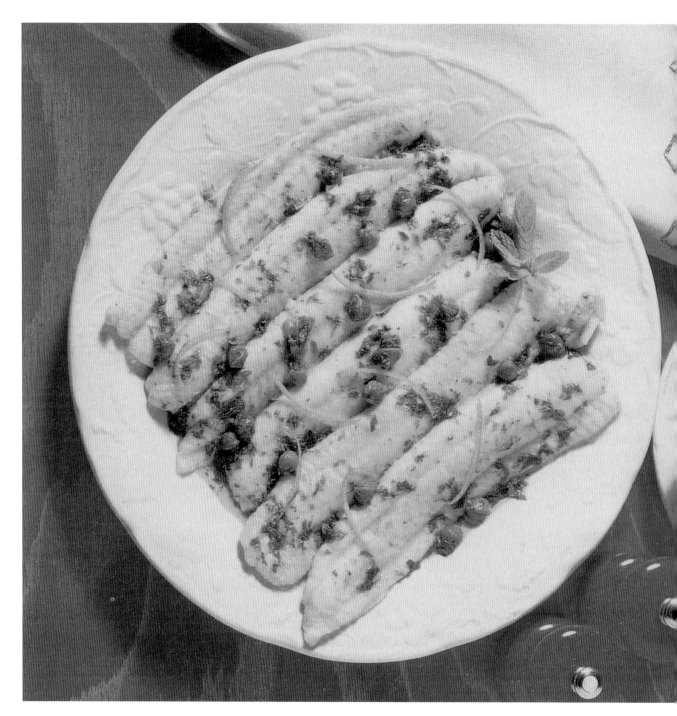

Steamed fish and herbs

Tangy Citrus Liver

1 calf's liver, peeled and dried
2 onions, chopped
2 cloves garlic, chopped
Juices of 3 oranges plus a little grated rind
2 tablespoons wholemeal flour or 1 tablespoon of arrowroot

Method: Seal and cook the liver and onion gently in a little water in a wok or stainless steel pan. Add garlic, citrus juices and peel. Thicken with wholemeal flour or arrowroot.

Liver Loaf

1 large lambs fry
$\frac{1}{4}$ cup diced celery
2 tablespoons minced parsley
$\frac{1}{4}$ teaspoon paprika
1 tablespoon celery leaves, minced
4 tablespoons finely chopped green pepper
1 teaspoon mixed herbs, dry or chopped fresh
$\frac{1}{2}$ cup minced onion
$1\frac{1}{2}$ cups grated carrots
3 tablespoons fresh wheatgerm
2 free range eggs, beaten

Method: Put liver through finest mincing blade, followed by the vegetables. Combine all ingredients and mix thoroughly. Put mixture in a large casserole dish and distribute evenly. Cover and bake in moderate oven (325-350°F). Uncover for 15 minutes for browning. This mixture is delicious if used for pies and pasties or in potato pie. The vegetable pulp left from making juices can be used in this loaf.

Kidney Paté or Spread

250 gms calf kidney, cooked and minced
1 raw onion, finely grated
¼ teaspoon dried marjoram or thyme
½ teaspoon vegetable seasoning
Yoghurt as required
4 tablespoons cottage cheese

Method: Blend all ingredients adding gradually enough yoghurt to make the mixture spread. Turn into screw top glass jar and chill. Keep refrigerated. Serve between leaves of lettuce or on potato, toast or rice crackers.

Liver Paté or Spread

½ lb liver, diced and trimmed of membranes and blood
  vessels
½ teaspoon vegetable seasoning
1 tablespoon arrowroot flour
1 chopped onion
Skim milk or stock as required
1 sprig parsley
Pinch of marjoram (oregano)
2 tablespoons pure water

Method: Heat water in pan searing liver on both sides lightly in it. Set aside. Sauté onion in same pan, cool. Put all ingredients one after the other into liquidiser adding enough stock to blend it into a smooth paste. Turn into small glass dish and chill. (If no liquidiser, this can be pounded to a smooth paste with a pestle and mortar).

Liver with Vegetables

Serves 4

3-4 tomatoes
250g (8 oz) liver, thin sliced
120g (4 oz) mushrooms chopped
1 stick celery chopped
½ teaspoon mixed chopped herbs
1 onion chopped
120g (4 oz) peas
1 medium sized carrot chopped
Vegetable stock if available or pure water

Method: Cook peas, onion and carrots in pure water. Drain off fluid to use as stock and put cooked vegetables in a covered casserole dish in the oven to keep warm.

Blend tomatoes and heat in stainless steel saucepan with stock saved from the vegetables. Add liver, mushrooms, celery and herbs and simmer for 10 minutes stirring occasionally.

Make a space in the centre of the cooked vegetables in the casserole and pile the liver mixture and juices into it.

Dot the vegetables with butter mixture, bread crumbs and cottage cheese. Put back in oven for 20 minutes or until topping melts and browns.

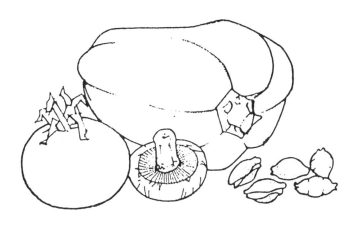

Baked Whole Fish

Serves 2

2 whole bream (individual fresh portion size approximately 300g)
2 tablespoons natural yoghurt
4 slices lemon
2 sprigs rosemary, bruised
2 springs lemon thyme, bruised
2 sheets butcher paper

Method: Ensure fish has been cleaned thoroughly. No need to remove scales. Spread some yoghurt inside each fish and place in lemon slices and herbs.

At this stage they can be left in the refrigerator to allow the flavours to penetrate the fish if time permits.

Wrap each fish individually in butchers paper to form a neat parcel. Wet each parcel with cold water until thoroughly soaked (but take care not to disintegrate the paper).

Place onto a baking slide and bake for 30 minutes at 200°C (400°F). Vary time according to size of fish.

When cooked, carefully remove paper. The scales and skin will stick to the paper and you are left with a beautiful, moist, tasty fish.

Serve with a large mixed salad. It can be served hot or cold. If to be served cold leave in paper so that skin keeps in juices and flavour until required.

Large fish can also be cooked in the same way and proportions cut off as required. Cold fish is ideal served with salad for lunch or dinner and a small portion makes an ideal breakfast dish.

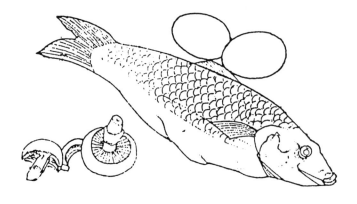

Spinach and Rice Pie

Pastry
1 cup wholemeal plain oaten flour
1 cup stone ground wholemeal wheaten flour
4 to 5 tablespoons iced water

Filling
3 cups chopped spinach
2 shallots, chopped
$\frac{1}{4}$ teaspoon nutmeg
$\frac{1}{2}$ cup cottage cheese
$\frac{1}{4}$ cup brown rice cooked
1 small tomato, diced
1 egg beaten

Method: To prepare pastry

Mix flours together in a large bowl. Add water a little at a time kneading well until dough is soft and flexible.

Wrap in plastic and refrigerate for 30 minutes.

Press pastry into greased 23cm quiche dish. Prick base all over with fork. Line dish with greased paper. Fill with dried beans or rice (bake blind). Bake in a moderately hot oven 190°C for 12 to 15 minutes or until golden. Remove beans (rice) and paper. Allow to cool.

To prepare filling

Steam spinach, shallots and nutmeg together until wilted. Drain. Combine with remaining ingredients.

Pour into pastry case. Bake in a moderate oven 180°C for about 25 minutes, or until set. Serve with a mixed salad.

Three Bean Pie or Loaf
(Gluten Free)

See page 21 for cooking hints for beans

Serves 4

½ cup ground millet or ½ cup ground rice
½ cup **cooked** kidney beans
½ cup **cooked** chickpeas
½ cup **cooked** green beans cut in 1 inch pieces
½ cup **chopped** onion (1 medium)
1 cup fresh mushroom
1 cup **cooked** soy beans
1 large ripe tomato
1 teaspoon 100% vegetable seasoning
1 small sprig of fresh basil
1 small sprig of fresh oregano or 1 teaspoon of dried herbs

Method: In a 'stick-free' pan, cook chopped onion in a small amount of water stirring for one minute. Add the mushroom and cover the pan, turn heat on low and simmer for another few minutes. Turn off the heat and keep pan covered while you prepare the rest of the recipe.

Into a blender put diced and peeled tomato, a few fresh basil and oregano leaves, 1 teaspoon of Bernard Jensen or other 100% vegetable seasoning and cooked soybeans. Blend until very smooth. Add ground millet or ground rice, cooked chickpeas, kidney beans and green beans.

Line a nine inch pie plate or a rectangular cake tin with oven paper. Pour the mixture in and bake in a moderate oven 350°F for 30 to 40 minutes.

Cut into segments or slice to serve.

Vegetables

For a meal select up to 5 vegetables including 1 green leafy,
1 red or yellow, 1 starchy such as potato or pumpkin.
Use a wide variety throughout the day especially in salads
and juices

Methods of preparation:

Scrub or wash all vegetables well to remove any dirt or residues.

Bake without oil, if necessary place on top of moist vegetables to prevent sticking. Leave skin on potatoes and pumpkin.

Boil in a minimum amount of purified rain water until tender (keep the water for soup stock).

Stir cook in pan with 2 tablespoons water. After initial searing cover to keep steam in and cook until tender on low heat.

Cooking in alfoil is quite safe if you wrap all the vegetables together with the shiny side in and the edges and ends folded up so that all the juices are contained. The package can be put in the oven, on the BBQ or under the griller to cook.

Bean and Vegetable Pot

2 cups diced potato
1 cup sliced carrot
2 cups green beans
1 or 2 onions, sliced
2 cups cooked red kidney beans (see page 21)
$\frac{1}{4}$ teaspoon each oregano and rosemary
$\frac{1}{4}$ cup chopped parsley

Method: Place all ingredients except parsley in saucepan, including bean liquid and 2 cups of vegetable stock. Bring to the boil and simmer 20 minutes, adding extra water if necessary.

Stir in parsley before serving.

Lentil Shepherd's Pie

1 cup dry brown lentils
1 onion, chopped
1 cup chopped carrots
1 cup diced celery
1 or 2 tomatoes
1 small capsicum, chopped
Herbs (perhaps $\frac{1}{4}$ teaspoon each sage, rosemary and
   oregano)
Crushed garlic to taste
2 cups potatoes mashed with a little of the lentil stock
Chopped parsley

Method: Cook lentils and vegetables and herbs in water to cover, adding more liquid (water or maybe fresh tomato juice) if needed. When lentils are cooked, place mixture in baking dish and cover with potato mixed with parsley. Bake at 350°F for 30 minutes.

Potato Cakes

3 cups diced potato
1 onion, chopped
Handful of grated carrot
$\frac{1}{4}$ cup chopped parsley
$\frac{1}{4}$ teaspoon each sage and basil

Method: Steam potato and onion. Mix in other ingredients after mashing the cooked vegetables. Form into patties and bake on a tray lined with oven paper. Bake at 350°F for 30 minutes. Turn up heat a little to brown tops if needed. Any left over vegetables may be added for variation.

Curry Sauce with Vegetables

1 medium potato, chopped in large pieces
2 medium carrots, diced
2-3 zucchinis, chopped

For the sauce
3 large tomatoes, chopped
$\frac{1}{4}$ cup apple juice
1 onion, chopped
Crushed garlic to taste
$\frac{1}{8}$ teaspoon tumeric and cinnamon
$\frac{1}{4}$ teaspoon cummin and coriander

Method: Steam the vegetables until not quite soft. Cook onion and garlic in apple juice, uncovered. When most of the juice is gone, add the spices and stir. Add chopped tomatoes and cook on low heat until they are well cooked down. Add the steamed vegetables and stir. (Some extra liquid may need to be added if sauce too thick.)

Cover and cook for further 10 minutes, stirring frequently. Serve with salad or protein foods or as a main meal.

Tomato Topping or Paste

1 or 2 onions, sliced
Crushed garlic to taste
3 or 4 shallots, chopped
1 capsicum, diced
3 cups chopped tomato
1 teaspoon basil

Method: Simmer onions in small amount of water. Add other ingredients and simmer for 15 minutes.

Blend or mash and simmer longer to make tomato paste.

Kidney with Rice and Onions

9 lamb kidneys or one calf kidney
1 large onion, finely chopped
1 teaspoon mixed herbs
1 cup of washed brown rice
1 tablespoon of cold pressed olive oil
1 cup of vegetable stock

Method: Cut kidneys from the concave centre outwards, and remove the white fibrous tissue and fat. Dice them.

Sauté the rice, onion and kidney in a stainless steel or glass saucepan with the oil, stirring until all are coated.

Stir in 1 or 2 cups of stock, fit the lid and bring to boiling. Turn down the heat and stir occasionally. Simmer for $\frac{1}{2}$ to $\frac{3}{4}$ of an hour, or until the rice has taken up most of the stock.

If there is too much fluid, cornflour or arrowroot could be used to thicken.

Garnish with slices of fresh tomatoes and serve with green beans, brussel sprouts, carrots and corn on the cob. Also on toast, kidneys make an excellent breakfast or luncheon dish.

Vegetable Casserole

1 potato, thinly sliced
½ small sweet potato, thinly sliced
½ onion, thinly sliced
1 tomato, thinly sliced
1 cup chopped silverbeet
1 cup any other finely chopped or sliced vegetable or pulp
    left over from juicing
Juice of ½ lemon
Pinch mixed herbs

Method: Layer ingredients in casserole dish, finishing with tomato. Sprinkle with lemon juice and herbs, cover tightly and bake at 375°F to 400°F for 1 hour or until food is soft.

Zucchini and Carrot Pulp Patties

1 zucchini grated
3 cups of grated carrot or pulp left over from juicing
1 medium onion grated or finely chopped
3 free range eggs, beaten
½ teaspoon mixed dried or fresh herbs
¾ cup wholemeal plain flour
¼ teaspoon kelp powder (optional)

Method: Mix all ingredients together, form into patties, roll in wheatgerm then flatten. Cook on a hotplate or non-stick pan until brown on both sides. Serve with homemade tomato sauce (see page 102).

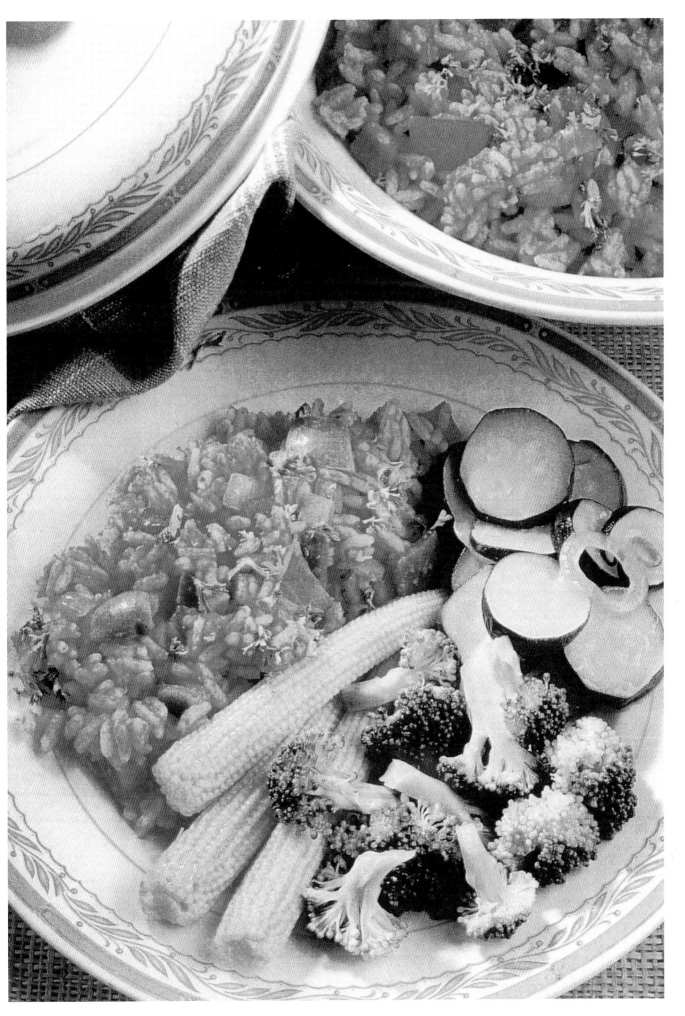

Rice and vegetables

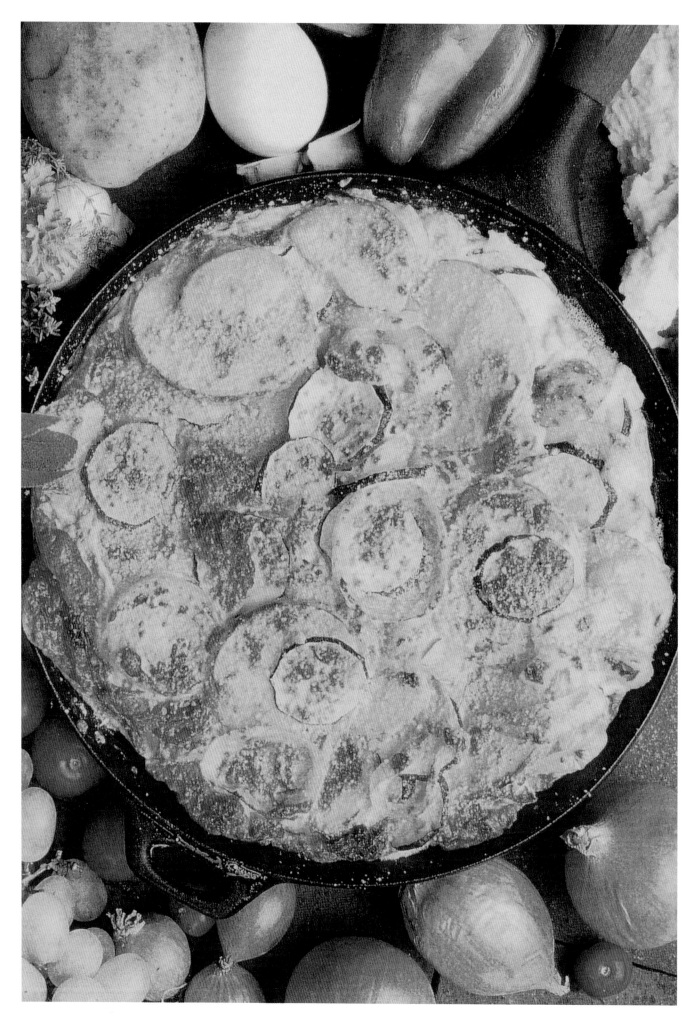

Quiche in a cast iron pan

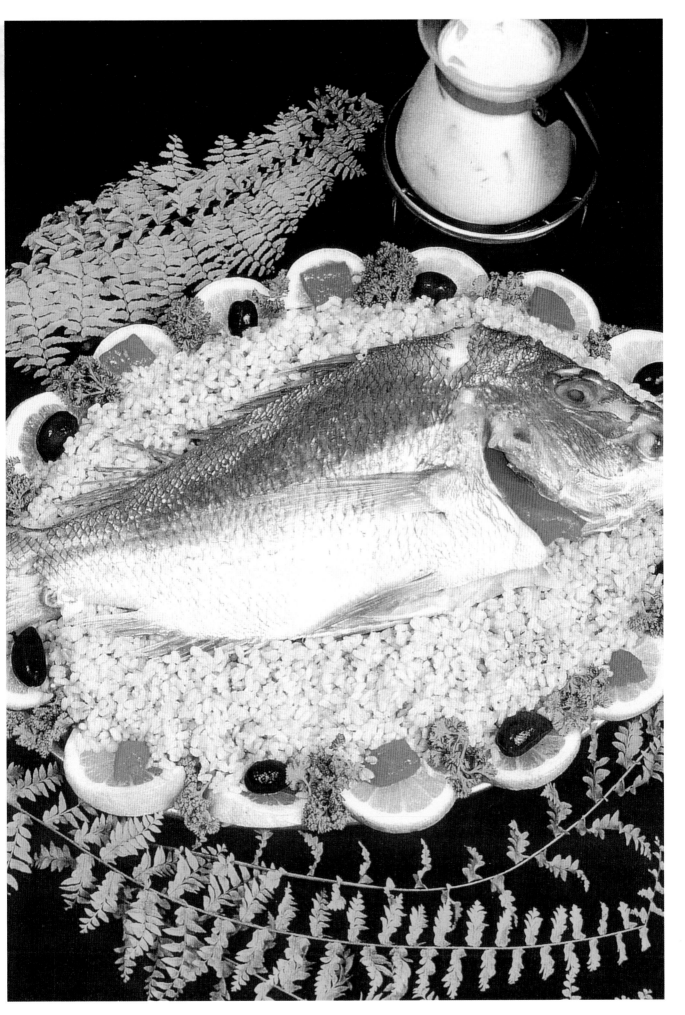

Baked whole fish with brown rice

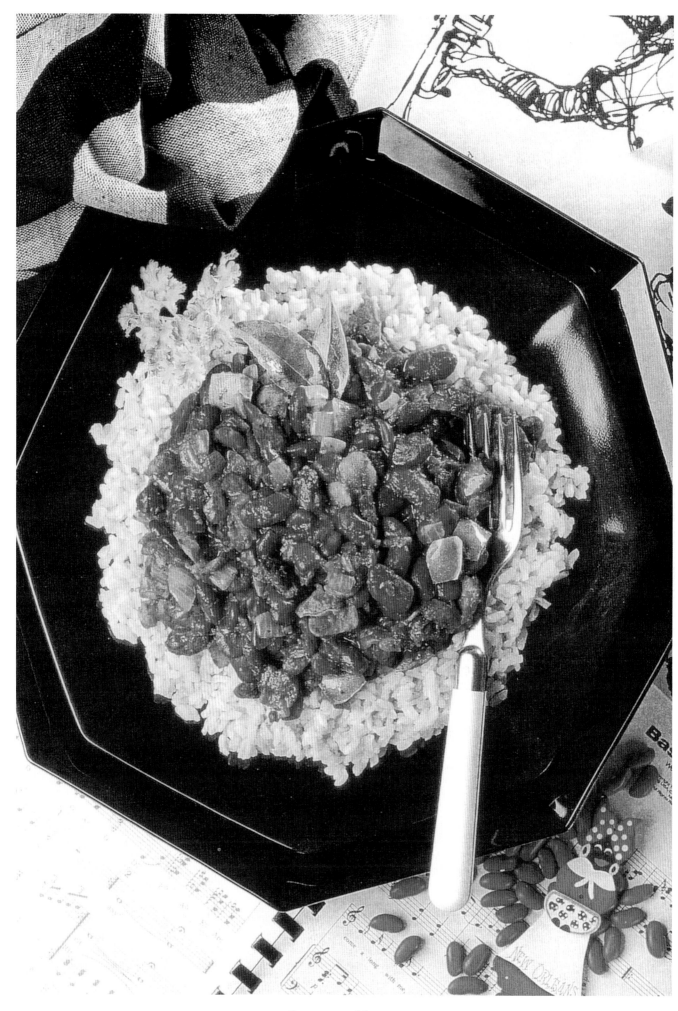

Bean vegetable pot

Desserts

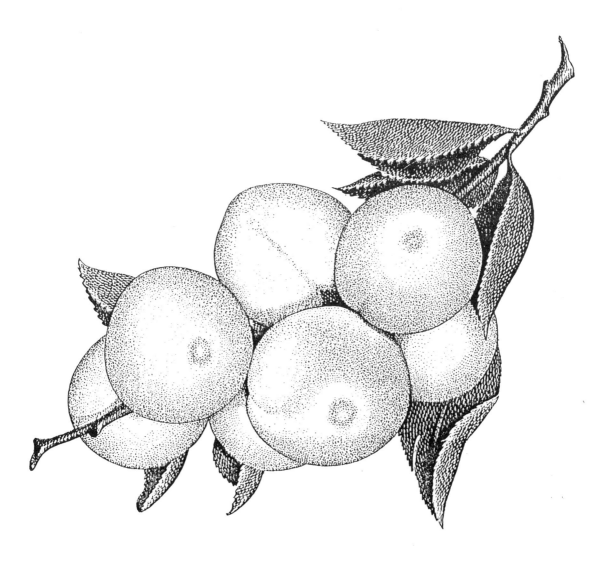

Carrot Muffins

1 cup grated carrot
1 cup grated apple
1 cup rolled oats
$\frac{1}{2}$ cup wheatgerm
$\frac{1}{4}$ cup rice flour
$\frac{1}{4}$ cup sunflower seeds
2 tablespoons cold pressed Linseed or C.P. Safflower oil
$\frac{1}{2}$ cup apple juice

Method: Mix all ingredients together with sufficient apple juice to form a soft mixture. With a dessertspoon form the mixture into balls and place on a baking tray. Flatten each ball slightly.

There is no need to oil the baking tray, as the oil in the muffins prevents them from sticking.

Bake at 170°C (340°F) for 25 minutes. This gives a nice soft muffin. If a crisper result is preferred bake for a little longer.

Makes approximately 20.

Ginger Baked Pears

Serves 2

2 pears
Raisins
2 teaspoons finely grated green ginger
$\frac{1}{2}$ cup apple juice

Method: Wash pears thoroughly. Remove core from the base of each, leave stem intact.

Fill each pear with raisins and a little green ginger. Place pears in an ovenproof dish, pour in apple juice and remaining ginger.

Bake in the oven at 200°C (400°F) for about 30 minutes, or until tender.

Serve warm or cold with pear cream or yoghurt. (See page 63.)

Pear Cream

¼ cup natural yoghurt
1 pear, peeled and cored
8 raisins, chopped (optional)

Method: Place all ingredients into a blender basin and blend until smooth.

Serve with desserts, such as ginger baked pears.

Other fruits can be used instead of the pear. Banana cream is delicious with fresh fruit salad or strawberries.

Pawpaw and Banana Sauce

1 cup pawpaw, roughly chopped
1 banana, sliced
Juice ½ lemon

Method: This can be used raw or uncooked. Even if raw the lemon will stop the banana discolouring. To cook place all ingredients into a saucepan, cover and simmer for five minutes. Puree fruit and liquid together to make a sauce. Delicious spread over apple cake.

Substitute any other fruits such as apricots, peaches or rockmelon.

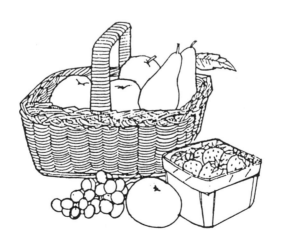

Carrot and Date Loaf

2 cups wholemeal flour
1 teaspoon bicarb of soda
1 cup unprocessed bran
$\frac{1}{4}$ teaspoon ginger powder or grated ginger
$1\frac{1}{4}$ cup Carnation skim milk powder
$\frac{1}{2}$ cup (150g) chopped dates
2 cups carrots, cooked and mashed
2 free range eggs
2 tablespoons honey
$\frac{1}{2}$-2 cups apple juice. Use your own judgement

Method: Combine the first seven ingredients in a bowl.

In a separate bowl whisk together remaining ingredients except juice. Stir together adding juice a little at a time to make a moist consistency. Put mixture in a lined loaf tin and bake in moderate oven 35 to 40 minutes.

Carrot and Banana Cake

2 eggs
1 cup grated carrot (or pulp from carrot/apple juice and
    some of the juice)
2 ripe bananas, mashed
$\frac{1}{4}$ cup cold pressed oil
$1\frac{1}{2}$ cups plain wholemeal flour
1 teaspoon bicarb of soda, (sieve together with flour)
$\frac{1}{2}$ teaspoon cinnamon
2 tablespoons of pure honey

Method: Beat eggs until light and fluffy. Add oil and honey and continue beating. Fold in carrot and banana and then add flour and cinnamon. Add further juice if needed so mixture is not too dry.

Bake 25 to 40 minutes at 180°C.

Apple Dessert Cake

2 slices of bread made into crumbs
2 apples peeled and sliced
5 fluid oz skim milk (use Carnation skim milk powder)
2 free range eggs
2 teaspoons lemon juice
Grated rind 1/2 lemon
2 tablespoons sultanas

Method: Cook apples in a stainless steel saucepan in a few drops of water with the lid on. Pour milk over breadcrumbs and leave to soak. Separate eggs and beat whites until stiff peaks form. Beat yolks until creamy. Add breadcrumbs, apple, lemon juice and rind and beat thoroughly. Fold in egg whites gently.

Pour into 6 inch cake tin. Bake at 180°C for 35-40 minutes. The cake is cooked when it springs back if pressed with finger. Turn it out to cool.

This cake may "drop" when cooling but still tastes great.

Apple Cake

3 green apples, peeled and diced into 1cm cubes
¼ cup raisins, finely chopped
1 cup wholemeal flour
½ cup oatmeal
2-3 oz apple juice
2 egg whites, whisked

Method: Combine first four ingredients together and add sufficient apple juice to make a moist mixture. Fold the whisked egg whites gently through the mixture.

Line a loaf container with greaseproof paper and place mixture in, smoothing off the top. Bake in the oven at 180°C (350°F) for 45-50 minutes. Cool slightly in tin before turning out. Top with pawpaw and banana slice.

Wholemeal Carrot and Sultana Cake

2 cups wholemeal stone ground flour
1 teaspoon baking powder (see page 00)
1 teaspoon mixed spice
1 tablespoon butter mixture (see page 00)
1 egg (free range)
1 cup skim milk
1 tablespoon honey
1 cup very finely grated carrots
1 cup natural sultanas, washed

Method: Sift flour, baking powder and spices, into a bowl. Rub in a special butter mixture till crumbly. Beat together egg, milk, honey and add to dry ingredients. Add carrot and sultanas. Stir only until just combined. Do not over mix. Put into foiled loaf tin. Bake in moderate slow oven 325°F for approximately 45 minutes.

Cooked mashed pumpkin can be used instead of carrot for variety.

Christmas Cake

370g green apples cooked
125g (½ cup) raisins
250g (1 cup) currants
250g (1 cup) sultanas
250g of butter mixture or 2 tablespoons of cold pressed flax oil
¼ cup honey
Rind and juice ½ orange
Rind and Juice 1 lemon
2 tablespoons of crushed almonds or macadamia nuts
½ teaspoon ginger
½ teaspoon cinnamon
½ teaspoon nutmeg

Method: Mix all above ingredients together and allow to stand in fridge overnight.

Then add:
1 teaspoon natural vanilla essence
8 oz wholemeal flour
½ teaspoon bicarb soda
3 eggs, beaten

Mix well and add more moisture if mixture is too dry. Cook approximately 1 hour in a moderate oven (180°C).

It keeps 4 weeks or more if wrapped in foil and placed in an air tight tin.

Apple Spice Cake

1 tablespoon honey
1 cup fresh apple sauce
¼ cup raisins
3 oz apple or grape juice
½ teaspoon allspice
¼ teaspoon mace
¼ teaspoon coriander
1½ cups oat flour
¾ cup wholewheat, triticale or other flour

Method: Combine honey and apple sauce. Sift all ingredients in and add raisins to the apple sauce. Pour into the non-stick oblong baking pan or pie dish. Mix crumb topping and sprinkle on top. Bake at 325°F for 40 minutes or until cake is cooked. Serve with a spoonful of apple sauce or non-fat yoghurt.

Crumb Topping

⅔ cup rolled oats or flaked rye
1 tablespoon honey
½ teaspoon allspice
Pinch mace

Method: Put oats, briefly in blender to make a finer flake. Mix spices with oats. Mix in enough sweetener to make a crumbly mixture. Sprinkle thickly on the Apple Spice Cake before cooking.

Strawberry Snow

Serves 4

250g strawberries
2 tablespoons arrowroot
2 tablespoons water
¼ cup natural yoghurt
2 egg whites

Method: Thoroughly rinse strawberries. Reserve four for garnish. Blend remaining strawberries to a smooth puree. Pass through a sieve to remove seeds if required.

Pour puree into a saucepan and bring to the boil. Mix arrowroot and water together, add to the strawberry puree and stir until thickened.

Pour into a bowl, leave to cool then stir in yoghurt.

Whisk egg whites to the soft peak stage. Fold through the strawberry yoghurt mixture.

Pour into a serving dish and chill before serving. Decorate with reserved fruit.

Other fruits can also be used when strawberries are out of season. Pawpaw makes a suitable alternative. Particularly delicious with a little passionfruit pulp mixed through.

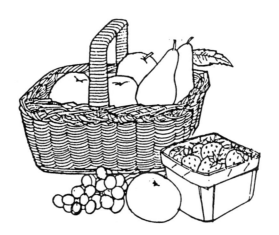

Banana Health Candy

4 bananas (cavendish are best)
¼ cup apple juice
10 chopped almonds or 15 apricot kernels
½ lemon, juice and grated rind
2 tablespoons wheatgerm
½ cup sultanas
½ cup dessicated coconut
Extra dessicated coconut for rolling

Method: Gently simmer bananas and apple juice in a covered saucepan until fruit is soft and most of the liquid has evaporated. Add remaining ingredients, except for extra coconut and mix well.

Divide mixture into four, shape each into a long roll approximately 15cm in length. Roll extra coconut around the outside of each one. Refrigerate for two hours or until firm before cutting into slices about 1cm thick.

Use as a sweet treat, but it is not intended for consumption in large quantities at once.

Note: Before grating rind from lemon, wash thoroughly to remove any residue.

Pawpaw, apricots and peaches can also be used instead of bananas when available. Apricots health candy is particularly delicious. This can be stored in the deep freezer for up to two months and used as required.

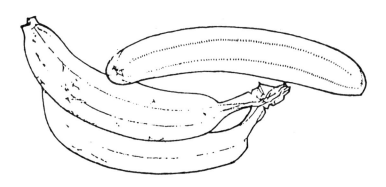

Frozen Fruit Dessert

1 litre concentrated fruit pureé or juice. Sweeten to taste
    with apple pureé or juice
Squeeze lemon juice
2 egg whites, whisked

Method: Sweeten fruit pureé if necessary with apple pureé or juice. Add a squeeze of lemon juice to bring out the flavour of the dominant fruit. Pour juice into a shallow freezer proof container.

    Place in deep freezer and freeze until semi-solid.

    Whisk egg whies to soft peak stage. Fold into semi-frozen juice. Pour mixture into a freezer-proof container with lid. Freeze until solid then serve for dessert with a selection of fresh fruits.

Note: Many fruits are naturally sweet enough not to require any additional sweetener from apple juice, for example, pineapples in the summer months are at their sweetest for those who can have them on the program.

Frozen Fruit

Ideal for that refreshing something during the hot summer months. Suitable fruits include grapes, bananas, peaches, pears, melons, pawpaws, etc.

Grapes   Break into small bunches of 3 or 4 grapes. Wash well and pat dry. Place on a try and freeze for approximately 1 hour. Remove when required.

Bananas   Place whole bananas with skin intact into deep freezer. Freeze for approximately 30 minutes to 1 hour or just firm. Remove skin and eat immediately.

Dried Fruit Leathers

Make a pureé of pure fruit.

Do not add any water or sweetener. If the fruit being used is likely to go brown such as bananas or apples, the pureé can be cooked before drying to prevent discolouration. Pour into a foil tray approximately $\frac{1}{2}$ cm thick and sun dry. Cover with muslin to prevent contamination and keep away from ants. They love it too.

Once it is firm, similar to leather, it can be cut into strips and rolled up. These make very tasty chews. It is recommended that these be stored in the refrigerator as the moisture content is too high to stop mould formation.

Any fruit can be dried to make leathers, the moisture content determines the drying period. The less moisture obviously the quicker it will dry.

Baked Apples

Core apples and stuff with dried fruit. Sprinkle with ground cloves, nutmeg or cinammon and place in an open casserole. Add $\frac{1}{4}$ inch apple juice and cook at 350°F until soft. Serve hot or cold.

Baked Bananas

Peel bananas, slice in half lengthwise if desired, and place in an open casserole with lots of juice. A mixture of pear and orange is tasty, or orange and apple. Sprinkle with nutmeg or cinnamon, or ground cloves, or a few crushed almonds or macadamias. Bake at 350°F until bananas are soft.

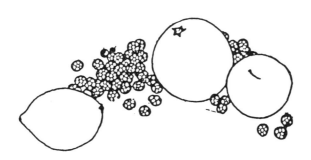

Apricot Spread

Take a pot full of fresh apricots whole or washed and dried
  halves
Juice of 1 or 2 oranges or $\frac{1}{2}$ cup of grape juice
Coarsely chopped ginger — as much as you like

Method: Mix ingredients in a stainless steel saucepan, bring to the boil quickly
with lid off. Simmer until soft with the lid on. Take pips out of whole apricots
when soft. Mash to make a thick sauce or spread.

Put in cut up macadamia pieces and washed raisins if liked.

Frozen Mush Patties

Take ingredients of already mixed muesli: wheatgerm, bran, dolomite, lecithin.
Add mashed banana to make into kneading consistencies. Add some of the
Apricot Spread with raisins. Form into patties. Roll in wheatgerm, seasame seeds
and coconut.

Freeze overnight. Use in the morning with yoghurt. May also have apples
stewed in orange juice with it.

Do not use this recipe if you have had a bypass operation for bowel cancer as
it contains a large amount of fibre.

Apple Pudding

1 teaspoon grated lemon rind
5 tablespoons of arrowroot
$\frac{1}{2}$ teaspoon honey
$\frac{1}{2}$ cup water
$1\frac{1}{2}$ cups real apple juice
1 large apple grated or diced fine
Cinnamon

Method: Stir the arrowroot into the $\frac{1}{2}$ cup of water. Add this mixture to the $1\frac{1}{2}$
cups of apple juice that has been brought to a boil, stirring over the heat until it
clears and thickens.

Remove from heat and add the remaining ingredients.

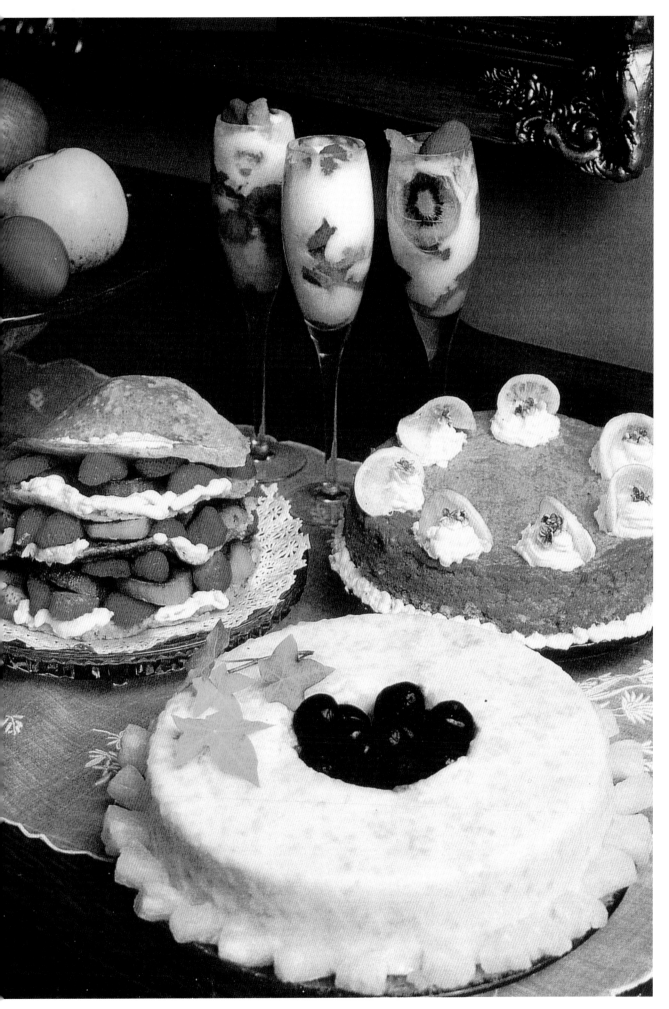

Pancakes and cakes

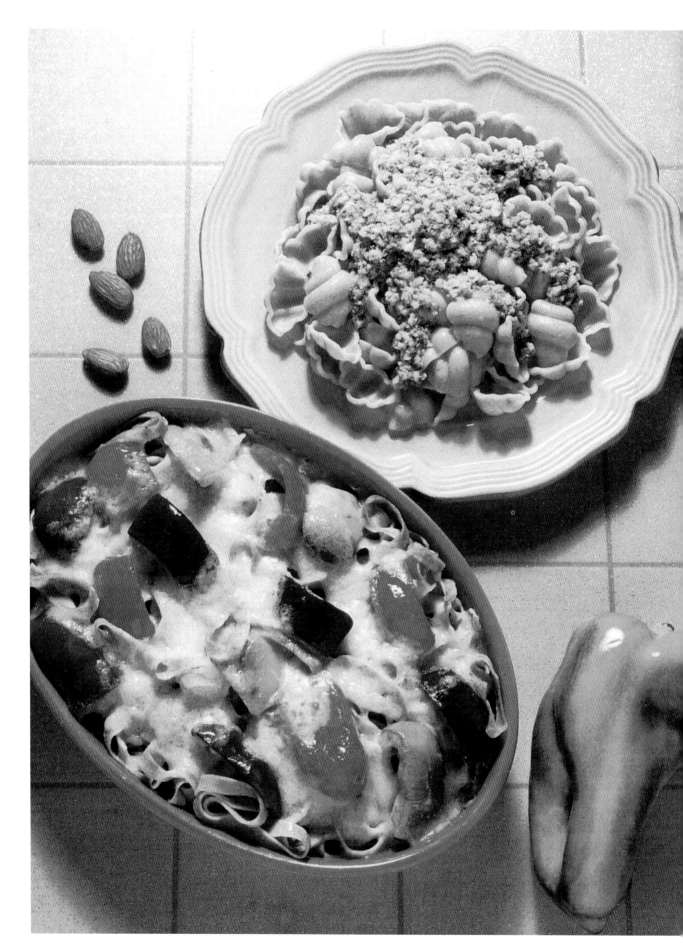

Wholemeal pastas

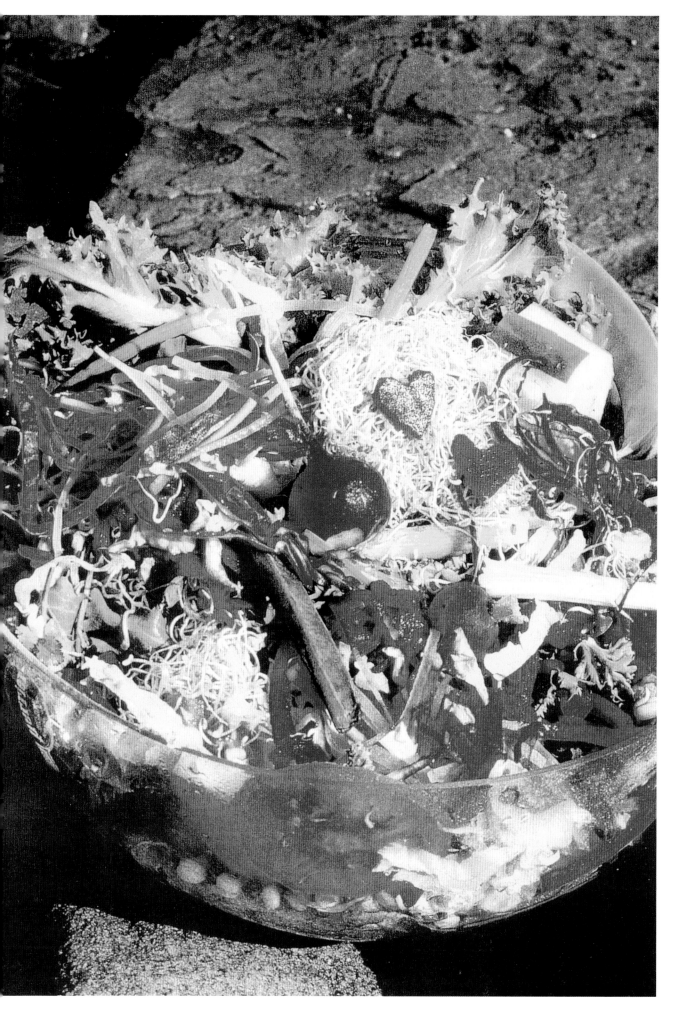

Grated salad

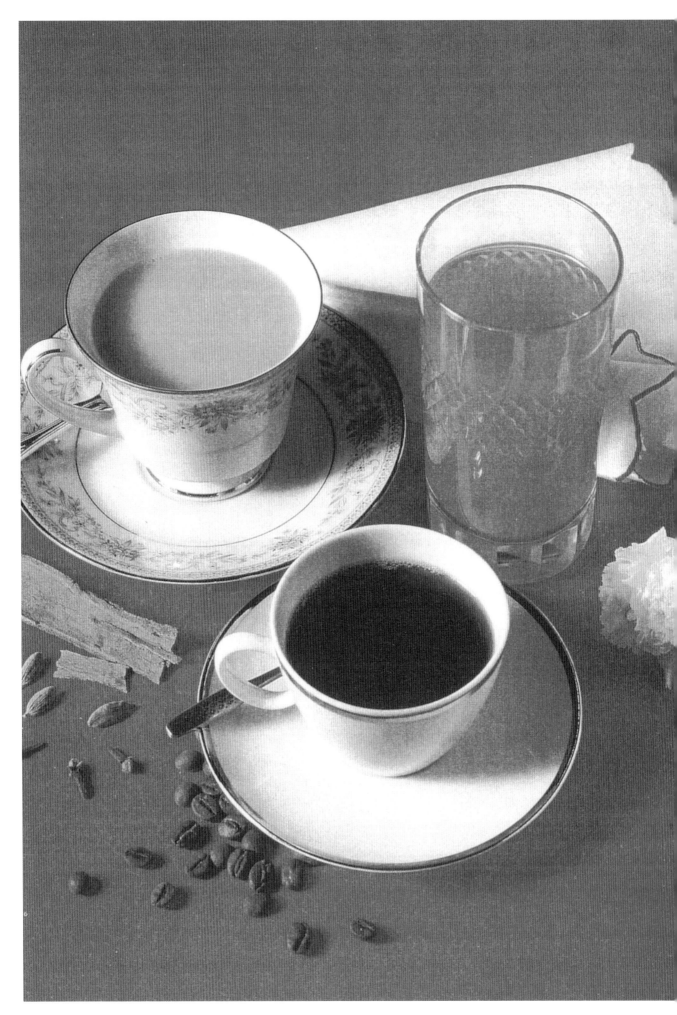

Herb teas

Figgy Pudding

$\frac{1}{4}$ cup figs, chopped
$\frac{1}{4}$ cup dates, pitted and chopped
1 teaspoon grated lemon rind
5 tablespoons arrowroot
$\frac{1}{2}$ cup water
$1\frac{1}{2}$ cups water, boiling

Method: Blend the figs and dates with enough water to make a thick spread, set aside.

Add the arrowroot into $\frac{1}{2}$ cup of water stirring until smooth. Add the arrowroot mixture to $1\frac{1}{2}$ cups of boiling water stirring it over the heat and allowing it to clear and thicken adding the fig, date mixture and rind little by little with yoghurt if desired.

Suggestion. If you wish to keep the fig, date mixture raw, you may add it and the yoghurt after the pudding has cooled.

Baked Custard

3 eggs
600ml skim milk
1 tablespoon honey
Vanilla bean or $\frac{1}{2}$ teaspoon of natural vanilla
Nutmeg

Method: Beat eggs well. Add milk. Pour into a greased ovenproof dish. Dribble honey over and stir. Add vanilla for flavour (optional). Sprinkle with nutmeg.

Stand in a baking dish of water and bake in a slow oven until set.

Bread and Butter Pudding

Add $\frac{1}{4}$ cup sultanas to custard mixture. Arrange thinly sliced triangles of buttered bread on top of custard. Make sure bread is saturated with custard before baking.

Honey may be reduced if sultanas are used.

Honey Pears

Serves 4

4 medium firm ripe pears
1 tablespoon honey
$\frac{1}{2}$ teaspoon ground ginger or cinnamon
$\frac{1}{2}$ cup water
Raw flaked almonds

Method: Peel, quarter and remove the cores from pears. Combine honey, spices and water in a large pan. Stir until the sauce boils. Add pears, cover and cook over very moderate heat, until syrup thickens to desired taste. Scatter almonds over.

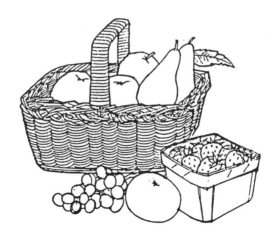

Pears in Orange Sauce

6 pears
1 tablespoon honey
¾ cup water
Juice of 2 oranges
Rind of 1 orange
Juice of 1 lemon

Method: Peel and halve pears. Place in ovenproof dish. Combine water, honey, juices and rind in a saucepan and heat until honey has melted. Pour over pears and cover. Cook in a moderate oven for 1 hour until pears are tender.

Tropical Sago

¼ cup sago
1½ cups orange juice
2 bananas
Few passionfruit

Method: Cook sago in juice and water for 10 minutes, stirring constantly over low heat. Add chopped bananas and pulp of passionfruit, and continue cooking until sago is clear, soft and thickened.

Fruit Rice

¼ cup rice
½ cup water
½ cup orange juice
Fresh fruit — banana plus pear and/or apple, few stewed
   prunes.
Sultanas may be added.

Method: Mix all together and bring to the boil. Simmer, stirring frequently to avoid burning, until rice is cooked. Cook until thick.
   Serve hot or cold, adding yoghurt if your diet permits.

Creamy Rice with no Milk

1 cup brown rice
3 cups water
2 chopped bananas
6 prunes
3 pieces diced pear
1 diced apple
1 cup orange juice

Method: Mix together and bring to the boil. Cook carefully to avoid sticking and burning until the rice and fruit is cooked and soft. Continue cooking until the liquid level is reduced and a thick consistency is reached.
   Serve hot or cold. Adding yoghurt is nice if your diet permits.

Classical Rice Pudding

Serves 4

Rice pudding is a wonderfully warming and satisfying dish and is almost a meal in itself.

    3 oz (85g) short grain brown rice
    1 pt (0.6 lt) skim milk
    2 teaspoons runny honey
    Few drops natural vanilla essence
    Nutmeg to taste

Method: Soak the rice in cold water for at least $\frac{1}{2}$ hour. Drain and rinse. Put into a pudding dish with the milk, honey and vanilla essence. Sprinkle on grated nutmeg. Bake in an oven at 350°F (gas3) for about 2 hours till the rice is soft and has absorbed most of the milk. You may have to top up the milk.

   Washed, soaked and chopped dried apples, pears, prunes or apricots may be cooked with the rice or stewed fruit may be served with it.

Sweet Tart Shell *(wheat free)*

    $\frac{1}{2}$ cup brown rice flour
    $\frac{1}{2}$ cup tricale flour
    $\frac{1}{2}$ cup oat bran or oat flour
    $\frac{1}{4}$ cup finely grated coconut
    Real grape or apple juice

Method: Mix dry ingredients well, add a little juice at a time kneading well to make a soft flexible dough.

   Press pastry into paper-lined tart or quiche dish.

   Bake in a moderate oven 12–15 minutes or until golden brown. Allow to cool undisturbed.

Blended Ice Cream

Serves 4

1 cup of ripe pawpaw, diced
4 bananas, frozen
1 mango, diced
Any other fruit, sliced
1 cup of skim milk yoghurt (optional)

Method: Peel and freeze four bananas. Place in food processor or blender with pawpaw and other ingredients. Put on "puree" or "whip" gauge and process, turning machine on and off until blended into a smooth ice-cream.
   Delicious!

Fruit Cream Dessert

280 ml natural low fat yoghurt
3 tablespoons skim milk powder
4 tablespoons unflavoured gelatine
1 to 2 cups of fruit (e.g. strawberries and/or peaches)
6 dried apricots and 1 tablespoon sultanas, washed and
     soaked may be used

Method: Put yoghurt, dried milk and gelatine in blender and blend for about 30 seconds.
   Add fruit, reserving some for decoration, and blend again. Pour into glasses and chill for 1 hour before serving.
   Makes two generous servings.

Bread & Pasta Recipes

Wholemeal Bread

500g stone ground wholemeal flour
50 - 60g gluten flour
2 sachets dried yeast or 30g compressed
1 teaspoon vitamin C powder
Approximately 450ml water at blood heat

Method: Mix dry ingredients together. (If using compressed yeast, have it at room temperature and crumble it into water. Mix well, ensuring the water is still at blood heat when combined). Add water and combine, then turn out onto floured surface.

Knead 5 - 10 minutes until elastic, then return to bowl and allow to rise in a warm place, covered lightly with a tea towel, until double in bulk. Punch down and knead 1 minute. Allow to rise until again doubled in bulk and a finger indentation remains. Half fill greased bread baking tins.

Cook in hot oven (electric 230°C or 450°F, gas 190°C or 375°F) for 35 minutes. When cooked the loaf sounds hollow when tapped on its base.

Cool on wire rack.

Unleavened Bread

2 cups plain wholemeal flour of wheat, buckwheat, rye,
   oatmeal. (All give a different flavour or texture. Rye flour
   makes a good crisp bread ideal for dips. Wholemeal wheat
   flour makes a softer bread).
1 tablespoon butter
1 teaspoon cold pressed linseed or cold pressed safflower oil
½ to ¾ cup skim milk or buttermilk (Carnation skim milk
   powder reconstituted)

Method: Place flour into a bowl. Rub in butter and oil. Add sufficient milk to mix to a firm dough. Lightly knead until smooth.

Divide dough into 10 pieces. Roll out each piece into a thin circle on a well floured board. Stack onto a plate and cover with plastic wrap. At this stage they can be stored in the refrigerator and cooked individually as required.

To cook, pre-heat a non-stick frypan on high. Cook one at a time and lightly brown on each side.

Line a bread basket with a cloth serviette and place in flat breads as they are cooked. Fold edges of napkin over to keep them warm.

Delicious warm but equally as good cold if preferred.

The uncooked bread will keep in the refrigerator for 2 or 3 days before cooking. For long term storage place in deep freezer, then you have a permanent supply when required.

Butter Mixture

½lb (250g) ordinary butter (not salt reduced)
¾ cup cold pressed linseed (flax) or cold pressed safflower oil

Method: Chop butter up in a bowl and stand it in the sun or in a just warm oven until it is partly melted. Add the oil and beat with a fork or blender until smooth. Pour into a dish with lid and refrigerate to set. This butter mixture can be used in place of butter but is best for health if not cooked.

Wholegrain Flour Flat Bread

Makes 48 slices

1 quart buttermilk
6 cups whole flour (wheat, oat, rye, buckwheat or millet flour)

Method: Gradually add buttermilk to 3 cups of wholewheat flour, beat thoroughly stirring until dough leaves sides of bowl. Roll on lightly floured surface until nearly paper thin. Lift carefully onto greased cookie sheets. Bake at 375°F for 12 minutes until brown and crisp.

Serve hot.

Rye Flat Bread

Makes 16 slices

2 cups rye flour
¾ cup non-fat skim milk powder (Carnation)
¼ cup sesame seeds
¼ cup sunflower seeds (optional)
¼ teaspoon salt or "Pressor K" potassium salt
1 cup water
1 egg, well beaten

Method: Combine rye flour, dry milk, sesame seeds, sunflower seeds and salt, mix well. Stir in 1 cup water, mix well. Fold in egg.

Spoon out evenly on well greased and floured baking sheet. Flatten ⅓ to ½ inch thick with oiled hands. The dough will be very sticky.

Bake at 450°F for 10 to 12 minutes. Brown under broiler.

Best if served hot.

Homemade Whole Wheat Pasta

Basic homemade pasta with variations will make any shaped or flat noodle from whole wheat flour, with or without eggs, with complementary soy powder if desired, or even with spinach for green noodles.

Makes 4 to 6 servings

2 cups whole wheat flour
½ teaspoon vegetable seasoning
2 eggs
½ cup water

Method: Mix the flour and seasoning in a mound on a very clean board or counter. Make a well in the mound and break the eggs into it. Add a little water to the eggs, then beat them with a fork for 1 or 2 minutes, gradually drawing the flour from the well, adding the rest of the water a bit at a time.

Working with the palms, squeeze the mixture together until a crumbly paste is formed. Start kneading the dough, folding it over and over until it is well mixed, smooth and elastic, for 10 to 15 minutes. (If the dough remains too dry and flaky, add more water, only a tablespoon at a time. If it stays too wet, gradually knead in more flour by the tablespoon).

When the dough has become shiny, smooth and elastic, cover it with an inverted bowl or put it in a plastic food storage bag and allow it to rest for ½ hour.

Divide the dough into two or four sections on a lightly floured board. Roll each piece of dough as flat as possible with a sturdy rolling pin. Start from the centre of the piece and work out. Roll the dough lengthwise, turn, then roll crosswise. Repeat until the dough is as thin as possible — ⅛ inch or less. (To prevent the dough from sticking to the board, carefully lift it and sprinkle a little more on the board.)

Thinly rolled pasta may now be cut into various widths or shapes. For lasagne noodles, cut strips 1½ inches wide and about 12 inches long. For fettuccine, make narrow strips ⅛ to ¼ inch wide. (Fold the pasta strips accordian-style or roll them up as if you were rolling paper, then shred with a sharp knife at the desired interval for the width of noodles you need.)

You can also cut 4 and ¼ by 5 inch rectangles to make flat cooked noodles for stuffed rolled manicotti or cannelloni (instead of using crepes). You can cook the pasta immediately while it is still fresh, or air dry it on clean towels or hanging over a clothes horse. Uncooked noodles may be refrigerated in an airtight container for several days, or they may be frozen.

Cooking

To cook fresh pasta, drop it into boiling water, using about twice the volume of water as the amount of pasta. Allowing the pasta to simmer gently is best for preserving the nutrients than hard boiling. (Using less water means less dissolving of vitamins and minerals.) Cover the pot and stir several times during the simmering.

The pasta will take 8 to 10 minutes to cook al dente, or still firm enough to bite. Larger pieces take longer. Dried fresh pasta may take longer also, so time and test it by biting.

Variations

Whole Wheat and Pea Flour Pasta. Substitute 1 cup natural pea flour for 1 cup whole wheat flour.

Whole Wheat and Spinach Pasta. Substitute $\frac{1}{2}$ cup of pureéd or cooked spinach for water in the recipe.

Eggless Whole Wheat Pasta. Substitute 2 tablespoons of oil for egg and add $\frac{1}{4}$ cup more of water.

Eggless Whole Wheat and Pea Pasta. Use $1\frac{2}{3}$ cups whole wheat flour and $\frac{1}{3}$ cup natural pea powder. Use 2 tablespoons oil instead of eggs, and increase water to $\frac{2}{3}$ cup.

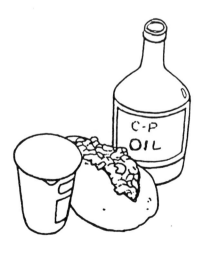

Muffins

2 cups wholemeal flour
2 teaspoons baking powder
1 cup skim milk (liquid)
1 cup washed raisins or dates
1/2 teaspoon ground ginger
1 teaspoon cinnamon
2 eggs
2 cups chopped apples (or any other fruit, blueberries are good)

Method: Preheat oven to 350°F (175°C).

Mix dry ingredients together.

Blend raisins or dates with milk.

Beat eggs, add apple or other fruit. Add to dry ingredients and mix thoroughly together. Place into non-stick muffin tins.

Bake for approximately 25 minutes reducing heat by 50°F in the last 10 minutes. Place on rack to cool.

Baking Powder

It is best to avoid any baking powder that contains aluminium salts since research has shown that aluminium can accumulate in the brain causing loss of memory and brain deterioration.

This is a suitable baking powder that can be easily made from the recipe that comes from the Rodale Test Kitchen.

2 tablespoons cream of tartar
2 tablespoons arrowroot
1 tablespoon baking soda

Method: Mix the ingredients together in a small bowl with a wooden spoon, crushing any lumps. Store in a tightly covered jar in a cool dry place.

Banana Nut Muffins

1¼ cups wholewheat flour
2 tablespoons honey
2½ teaspoons baking powder (see page 84)
½ teaspoon salt
¾ cup oats
1 egg, beaten
3 tablespoons cold pressed oil
½ cup milk
1 cup mashed very ripe bananas
⅓ cup chopped nuts

Method: Combine flour, baking powder, salt and oats. Add egg, oil, milk, honey, bananas and nuts. Stir only until dry ingredients are moistened. Fill greased muffin cups ⅔ full. Bake at 400°F for 15 minutes or until cooked through when tested with a skewer.

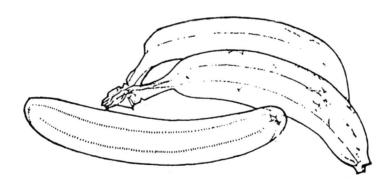

Wholegrain Pumpkin Muffins

Makes 12

$1\frac{1}{4}$ cups wholewheat flour
$\frac{1}{2}$ cup wheatgerm
2 tablespoons honey
$2\frac{1}{2}$ teaspoons baking powder (see page 84)
$\frac{1}{2}$ teaspoon salt (optional)
$\frac{1}{4}$ teaspoon ground cinnamon
$\frac{1}{4}$ teaspoon ground nutmeg
2 eggs
$\frac{3}{4}$ cup milk
$\frac{1}{2}$ cup pumpkin, cooked and mashed
$\frac{1}{4}$ cup cold pressed oil

Method: Stir together the flour, wheatgerm, baking powder, salt, cinnamon and nutmeg. Make a well in the centre. Combine egg, honey, milk, pumpkin and oil. Add all at once to dry ingredients. Stir until just moistened.

Spoon into greased muffin cups. Bake at 400°F for 15 to 20 minutes.

Pumpkin Scones

3 cups diced pumpkin, cooked and mashed
3 tablespoons butter mixture
3 cups of wholemeal flour (use wheat, oats or rye)
1 beaten egg

Method: Add butter to hot mashed pumpkin and let it cool.

Add the beaten egg and then the flour to make the consistency of a scone dough.

Cut into 2 inchs squares, place on a floured scone tray and bake at 400–410°F for about $\frac{1}{4}$ hour.

Poppy Seed Biscuits

Makes 8 dozen crackers

$\frac{1}{3}$ cup poppy seed
2 cups wholewheat flour
$\frac{1}{2}$ teaspoon salt (optional)
$\frac{1}{3}$ cup cold pressed oil
1 tablespoon honey (optional)
1 egg, slightly beaten
$\frac{1}{3}$ cup minced onion

Method: Combine poppy seed with $\frac{1}{3}$ cup boiling water. Cool. Place flour and salt into a bowl. Stir in remaining ingredients and poppy seed mixture, mixing well. Knead lightly on a floured surface until smooth.

Roll out half the dough at a time to $\frac{1}{8}$ inch thickness. Cut with $1\frac{1}{2}$ inch biscuit cutter or cut into squares. Place on baking sheet, prick with fork. Bake at 425°F for 10 minutes or until lightly browned. Store in an airtight container.

Pastry

Note on liquids: Tomato, onion or apple juice can be used as the liquid for pastry depending on whether a savoury or sweet pie is to be made. These are particularly good in the Tofu pastry.

Oatmeal and Pumpkin Pastry

2 cups oatmeal (or 3 cups rolled oats, processed to a fine meal)
2 cups mashed pumpkin
Pinch nutmeg
Water if necessary

Method: Mix oatmeal, pumpkin and nutmeg together to form a soft pastry. If necessary add extra water. This quantity will be adequate for a 22cm pie dish. If mixture is too soft to roll out, press out by hand and spread over the top layer with a knife. Mark the edge with a fork. This makes a very soft pie crust with good flavour.

Tofu Pastry

2 cups wholemeal flour
100g Tofu
½ cup water

Method: Mix flour and tofu together with fingers. Add sufficient water to form a stiff dough. This quantity will be adequate for a 22cm pie dish. This pastry is quite crisp with a pleasant flavour from the flour. It is excellent pastry to use for pies to be eaten cold.

Tofu and Pumpkin Pastry

2 cups wholemeal flour
100g Tofu
*¼ to ½ cup mashed pumpkin
Pinch nutmeg
½ cup water
*The quantity of pumpkin used depends on personal
   preference. The more added the softer is the final product,
   and the deeper the orange colour.

Method: Mix flour and tofu together with fingers, then add pumpkin and nutmeg.

Add sufficient water to form a soft dough.

For those on the Gerson program, Tofu (soy bean curd) can be replaced with cottage cheese or yoghurt. Adjust the water required accordingly. The yoghurt gives rather an acidic flavour to the pastry but this goes well with a fish and silverbeet filling.

Salads and Salad Dressings

Carrot and Nut Salad

3 carrots grated
2 teaspoons poppy seeds
6 macadamia nuts, chopped
1 tablespoon yoghurt
Sqeeze lemon juice

Method: Mix all ingredients together and chill well before serving. The flavour improves if refrigerated overnight. Apple or 2 teaspoons of sultanas can be added as a sweet lift to the salad if desired.

Watermelon Salad

500g watermelon, chopped, seeds removed
$\frac{1}{2}$ cup mung bean sprouts
$\frac{1}{2}$ cup cress, chopped
2 tablespoons basil, chopped

Method: Mix all ingredients together and chill well before serving.

Beetroot and Apple Salad

Grate equal quantities of beets (raw) and green apples as a side salad.

Coleslaw

Shred cabbage, carrot, celery, radish, zucchini, capsicum and green apple. Add orange juice, cold pressed safflower oil or mayonnaise. (page 97)
    Cooked brown rice may be added as an extra or substituted for the cabbage.

Grated Vegetable Salad

Grate equal quantities of carrot and zucchini. Add tomato dressing (see below).
An alternative dressing is apple and lemon juice, equal parts.

Tomato Dressing

½ cup fresh tomato juice
2 tablespoons lemon juice
1 tablespoon finely chopped capsicum or parsley

Method: Shake together and refrigerate.

Apple Sprout Salad

1 cup mung bean sprouts
1 cabbage, finely shredded
1 apple, finely chopped or shredded
Shredded radish for colour
¼ cup soaked raisins or sultanas

Method: Mix and use with Spicy Dressing.

Spicy Dressing

In the juice of a large lemon shake ¼ teaspoon each of ground cummin and
coriander and 1 teaspoon linseed oil or olive oil, cold pressed.

Chickpea Salad

3 teaspoons curry powder
1 teaspoon cummin seeds or powder
2 cups cooked chickpeas
1 or 2 zucchini, grated
1 carrot, grated
1 small onion, finely chopped
$\frac{1}{2}$ cup of washed currants or sultanas or raisins
$\frac{1}{4}$ cup chopped fresh parsley
$\frac{1}{4}$ cup lemon juice
Fresh herbs to garnish

Method: Heat water, add the onion, cook until translucent. Add curry powder and cummin. Stir well for 1 minute. Add chickpeas. Stir and cook until well coated in mixture.

Leave in a large bowl until cool. Add remaining ingredients. Garnish with fresh herbs.

Note: Chickpeas must be soaked overnight and cooked until soft before use. (See notes on cooking beans).

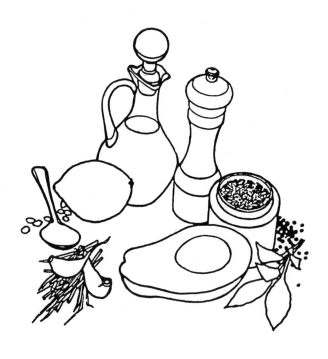

Fruit and Rice Salad

2 cups brown rice
1 orange
$\frac{1}{2}$ red capsicum, finely chopped
3 spring onions, sliced
1 green apple, peeled and finely chopped
$\frac{1}{2}$ cup walnuts or pecan nuts, chopped
$\frac{1}{4}$ cup slivered raw almonds
$\frac{1}{3}$ cup washed sultanas
$\frac{1}{3}$ cup chopped peaches or apricots
$\frac{1}{3}$ cup chopped dried pears
$\frac{1}{4}$ cup chopped fresh mint

Dressing

1 tablespoon grated fresh ginger
1 tablespoon lemon juice
1 cup apricot or grape juice
$\frac{1}{4}$ teaspoon ground cardamon

Method: Boil rice until cooked — rinse and drain.

Remove rind from orange with a vegetable peeler. Cut rind into thin pieces about 3 to 5cm long. Combine the dressing ingredients in a screw top jar and shake well. Mix all ingredients into rice, pour dressing over and mix well.

You can use some of the orange rind to garnish.

This recipe lends itself to variation so go ahead and experiment with different juices (orange with cinnamon is nice) and different spices including nutmeg.

You can also vary the combination of fruits and nuts.

Crunchy Salad

Grate quantities of carrot, peeled green apple, and celery chopped finely. Add orange juice to moisten.

The variety in your salads is only limited by your imagination. Try vegie fingers instead of grating for a change; tomato wedges instead of slices.

Be creative!

Red and Green Salad

1 head romaine or other green lettuce
2 cups savoy, or green or red cabbage shredded
3 green onions, sliced
1 cup sunflower greens
2 kohlrabi cut in shoe string strips, or use peeled broccoli
    stems or swede turnips
1 yellow squash, sliced thin
1 cup of cherry tomatoes or 1 large sweet red pepper cut in strips

Spinach Dressing

1 cup non-fat yoghurt
2 cups spinach chopped or 1 cup cooked spinach
3 green onions, chopped
1 to 2 teaspoons vinegar or lemon juice
$\frac{1}{2}$ teaspoon dill greens
Pinch mace (optional)

Method: Spin all ingredients in a blender until smooth.

Green Dilly Beans

3 cups green beans cut to 2 inch lengths
$\frac{1}{3}$ cup onion sliced in rings
$\frac{1}{2}$ teaspoon dill seed
2 tablespoons lemon juice

Method: Combine and bake in slow oven in a covered casserole until tender. Serve as a salad.

Sage and Sprouts Vegie Loaf

2 cups lentil sprouts
$\frac{1}{4}$ cup fresh parsley
$1\frac{1}{2}$ cups eggplant, diced finely or substitute parsnips or
    sweet potato
1 cup onions, chopped finely
$\frac{3}{4}$ cup beets, grated
$\frac{3}{4}$ cup carrots, grated
1 cup celery, chopped
3 cloves garlic, minced
$1\frac{1}{2}$ cups cooked brown rice
1 teaspoon thyme
$\frac{1}{2}$ teaspoon sage
$\frac{1}{4}$ teaspoon tarragon
1 tablespoon lemon juice
tomato sauce (page 102)

Method: Use two-day lentil sprouts. You'll want them to be a bit on the dry side so don't rinse them just before using. Grind sprouts, parsley and eggplant (or substitute) in a food grinder. Add remaining ingredients and mix well.

Bake in covered pan at 300-325°F for approximately $1\frac{1}{2}$ hours. Uncover and baste with sauce. Bake 10 minutes more at 375°F. Serve with extra sauce, cut in slices with salad.

Tabbouleh

$\frac{3}{4}$ cup burghul (cracked wheat)
1 small onion, finely chopped (optional)
$\frac{1}{4}$ cup chopped mint
$\frac{3}{4}$ cup chopped parsley
2 tomatoes, chopped
$\frac{1}{2}$ lemon, juiced
1 tablespoon cold pressed safflower or linseed oil
For variety sunflower sprouts are delicious in tabbouleh.

Method: Cover burghul with cold water and soak for 20 minutes. Drain burghul and pat dry.

Mix the burghul and the next 4 ingredients together in a salad bowl. Chill well. Just before serving shake the lemon juice and oil together then pour over the salad and lightly toss.

Tomatoes may be deleted for those having the herbal mixture.

Cottage Cheese Salad

Serves 2

1 cup cottage cheese
2 tablespoons natural yoghurt
$\frac{1}{2}$ cup mung bean sprouts
$\frac{1}{2}$ cup watermelon, finely chopped
2 shallots, chopped

Method: Lightly mix together all the ingredients. Chill well before serving. Serve with freshly made wholemeal unleavened bread.

For people with allergies to yeast use lemon juice instead of vinegar in salad dressings.

Herb and Buttermilk Dressing

In a blender mix together $\frac{1}{2}$ cup buttermilk and the herbs of your choice.

Suggestion. Mixed fresh herbs in buttermilk are delicious poured over a salad of sliced onion and tomato (or any other combination of salad vegetables). Dill is also delicious.

Oil and Vinegar Dressing

1 tablespoon cold pressed linseed or safflower oil
2 tablespoons lemon juice or apple cider vinegar

Method: Place oil and juice or vinegar into a screw top jar and shake well.
    Chopped herbs or garlic may also be added to complement the salad it is to be served with.

Mayonnaise

$\frac{1}{4}$ cup lemon juice or apple cider vinegar
2 tablespoons natural yoghurt
1 egg yolk
$\frac{1}{2}$ cup cold pressed linseed or safflower oil

Method: Blend the first three ingredients in a small bowl. Add oil while blending taking care not to curdle the mayonnaise by adding the oil too quickly.
    As a variation add chopped herbs, garlic or spices. This makes a lovely sharp mayonnaise, thin in consistency. Delicious poured over grated beetroot.
    If a thicker consistency is required use only 1 tablespoon of lemon juice or vinegar and 1 tablespoon of yoghurt.

Vegetable Snacks

Carrots
Cauliflowerettes
String Beans
Cherry Tomatoes
Zucchini
Turnips
Celery
Cucumber
Radishes
Tender Broccoli
Green Peas

Method: Arrange attractively for colour and flavour. Cut into shapes to eat with fingers — strips, rings, rounds, wedges, hearts, etc.

Serve any raw vegetables this way including watercress, lettuce and nasturtium leaves.

These vegetables may be arranged attractively on a platter, divided serving dishes, on a lazy susan or in separate containers.

Chickpea Spread

Rinse 1 cup of chickpeas.

Soak chickpeas overnight for 6 hours.

Cook in a stainless steel saucepan in pure water for 30-40 minutes.

Add raw washed sesame seeds and a crushed clove of garlic if liked. Blend well with a little water plus enough cold pressed linseed oil to make a paste. Add a tablespoon of yoghurt or some lemon juice.

This is a good spreadable paste for Rye Vitas, toast or pita bread.

Sauces etc.

Thick Tomato Sauce

3 tomatoes, chopped
1 red capsicum, chopped
2 shallots, chopped
1 peeled apple, chopped
¼ cup apple cider vinegar or lemon juice
Pinch cayenne pepper (optional)
1 sprig basil

Method: Place all ingredients into a saucepan. Bring to the boil and simmer for 30 minutes. Allow to cool slightly then process in a food processor to the desired consistency. Use as required. Store in sterilised jars.

Use as an accompaniment to fish, pies or pasta.

For people on a tomato free program this is still delicious without the tomatoes, use more capsicums if desired.

For those with an allergy to yeast use the lemon juice instead of the vinegar.

Capsicum Pureé

1 large red pepper
1 shallot
1 clove garlic
Sprig of mint
1 tablespoon apple cider vinegar or lemon juice
(Lemon juice is to be used for those with an allergy to yeast.)

Method: Process all ingredients together in a food processor to a fine consistency.

Pour into a saucepan and boil for 5 minutes. If a fine pureé is required blend the mixture or press it through a plastic sieve after cooking.

Vegetable Stock

1 onion, chopped
1 carrot, sliced
1 stalk celery, sliced
1 leaf silverbeet, sliced
4 sprigs parsley
1 sprig basil
4 garlic chives or 1 garlic clove and chives

Method: Place all ingredients into a saucepan and cover generously with water. Bring to the boil and simmer for 45 minutes. Strain and use as required.

Mango Chutney

2 dozen green or half ripe mangoes
2 granny smith apples
8 ripe apricots, pitted
375g or 1 packet of washed sultanas
1 nob or 8 cloves of raw garlic, peeled and chopped finely
3 large onions, peeled and chopped finely
1 cup of crystalised ginger, chopped fine
4 cups cider vinegar
2 cups white or red grape juice

Method: Cut the flesh off the mango seeds with a sharp knife and chop into small pieces across the grain of the fibres so that they do not make a large mat-like cotton wool when they have been cooked.

Similarly with apricots. Crack the apricot pits and add them to the large stainless steel saucepan.

If using preserved apricots they must be washed carefully to remove the metalisulphate before chopping them.

Peel and dice apples into the pan. Also add the onions, garlic, ginger, vinegar and grape juice. If fresh grape juice is not available the 100% concentrated bottled juice containing no added sugar or preservatives is satisfactory. Freshly extracted pear or apple juice is acceptable too for sweetness as there is no sugar in this recipe.

Mix well with a wooden spoon. Bring to the boil and turn heat down to simmer for 1 hour or until the fluid is reduced to a thick sauce consistency. Add more fruit juice if it becomes too thick. Stir with a wooden spoon to stop it catching.

Sterlise clean glass jars by heating them in the oven, also their lids, to 150°C for half an hour. Allow to cool in this oven to 'touch heat' while chutney is also cooling a little.

Fill jars completely, clean rims with fresh face tissue and screw down to seal lids on while still warm.

Mustard Sauce (1)

½ cup low fat unsweetened yoghurt
1 cup water or stock from vegetable, veal bone or turkey
¼ teaspoon thyme
1 teaspoon Dijon mustard
1 tablespoon wholemeal flour
6 mushrooms
4 spring onions

Method: Chop mushrooms and spring onions. Sauté in a little water. Thicken sauce with wholemeal flour adding stock, thyme and mustard. Hold for a day if possible. 1 teaspoon of curry powder instead of mustard may be used.

Mustard Sauce (2)

2 tablespoons water
½ pint water and 1 tablespoon cider vinegar
Lemon juice to taste
2 shallots peeled and chopped
1 tablespoon french mustard
2 tablespoons fresh chopped parsley

Method: Simmer shallots in water 1 minute. Add water/vinegar mix stirring constantly, allow mix to boil until reduced to ⅓. Remove from heat. Add mustard, lemon juice and parsley. Gently heat for a couple of minutes. Serve over liver. 1 teaspoon of curry powder instead of mustard may be used.

Mustard and curry sauces must not be hot. They should give the delicate taste without any irritation to the digestive tract.

Cucumber Dip

1 medium cucumber finely sliced or grated without seeds
3 shallots or some chives, finely chopped
1 clove garlic, crushed
½ teaspoon ground cummin
1 cup low natural yoghurt

Method: Combine all ingredients. Serve as a dip or a sauce.

Tomato Sauce

6 tomatoes
½ red capsicum, chopped
2 shallots or onion or chives, chopped
1 green apple, chopped
¼ cup apple cider vinegar or lemon juice
1 clove garlic
3 teaspoons of any fresh chopped herbs available, basil,
   oregano
2 sticks celery
2-4 teaspoons of vegetable seasoning

Method: Place all ingredients in stainless steel saucepan. Bring to the boil then simmer until tender. Cool then process through blender. Pour into muffin pan and freeze. Put into plastic bags and keep in freezer until needed.

Onion Gravy with Liver

Liver, sliced thinly and coated in wholemeal flour
1 onion, chopped
Water
3-4 teaspoons vegetable seasoning mix

Method: Simmer onion in little water until tender. Add seasoning mix and simmer further 2-3 minutes. Put through a blender and return to pan. Add liver and cook on low heat until cooked through, turn regularly and add water if gravy thickens too much.

Tomato Gravy

Use exactly the same recipe as above but omit the vegetable seasoning and add instead home made tomato paste (see recipe on page 57).

Marinade — Curry and Yoghurt

1 cup skim milk natural yoghurt
1 tablespoon lemon juice
1 tablespoon real orange juice
1 clove garlic, crushed
1/2 teaspoon curry powder

Method: Mix all together, pour over kebabs (see following recipe) in a shallow dish and marinate for 2 to 3 hours before grilling. What is left of the mixture may be spooned over the kebabs just before serving.

Variations

Apple cider vinegar may be used instead of the citrus juices.

1 teaspoon of grated fresh ginger or other fresh or mixed herbs such as shallots, oregano, basil may be added.

Kebabs

Almost any suitable vegetables and fruit may be cut into bite sized pieces and threaded onto a skewer.

Alternate different colours to make it look appealing and choose vegetables that will cook over the same time period when wrapped in foil; carrots, beans, onions, potatoes, celery and also pineapple, apple and banana. Faster cookers are tomato, capsicum, mushrooms and zucchini and cauliflower. When marinated place the kebabs on a foil sheet adding some of the marinade before sealing the package.

Cook on a barbeque plate or under the griller or in a fairly hot oven. Cooking will take about fifteen minutes.

Tofu Sandwich Filling or Dip

1 cup Tofu (soya bean curd)
2 cloves crushed garlic
$\frac{1}{2}$ onion, finely chopped
1 peeled tomato
1 tablespoon fresh parsley, chopped
1 tablespoon fresh basil, chopped
$\frac{1}{4}$ teaspoon dried thyme
$\frac{1}{2}$ teaspoon oregano

Method: Place all ingredients in food processor and blend until smooth. Have on fresh bread or Rye Vita or use as a dip.

Avocado Spread Dip

1 or 2 avocado depending on thickness required
Juice of $\frac{1}{2}$ lemon
$\frac{1}{4}$ cup mayonnaise (see recipe on page 97)
1 clove garlic
1 small onion
1 pinch kelp powder or "Bernard Jensen" seasoning

Method: Blend all together then chill.

Sprouts

Sprouting

A wide range of beans, grains and seeds can be sprouted to form a valuable addition to the diet.

Mung beans, lentils, barley, oats, fenugreek and sunflower are but a limited selection of those suitable for sprouting.

The directions given for sunflower seeds can be used for any other sprouts you wish to grow.

Sunflower Seed Sprouts

Cover sunflower seed with warm water and leave to stand for 6 hours. Place soaked seeds in a large necked jar. Cover with a piece of muslin and secure over opening. Leave in a light place, but away from direct sunlight.

Rinse the seeds daily by pouring water through the muslin and then turning the jar upside down on draining board to allow the water to drain away.

It takes 3 to 5 days for sprouts to grow depending on variety and length desired. Once sprouted, store in a refrigerator and use as soon as possible.

Sprouts Combination

1 cup washed sprouts
1 cup cottage cheese
1 diced avocado
$\frac{1}{4}$ cup low fat natural yoghurt
2 shallots or some chives, finely chopped
$\frac{1}{4}$ teaspoon kelp powder (optional)

Method: Fold all ingredients in together carefully without breaking up avocado or sprouts. Use as a side salad or as a filling for bread rolls, pita bread or crepes.

Milk Foods

Make Your Own Natural Yoghurt

¾ cup Carnation skim milk powder
500ml filtered water
1 tablespoon Pauls natural set yoghurt or ¼ teaspoon
    powdered lacto bacillus acidophilus

Method: Mix milk powder and water. Heat to lukewarm (40-46°C or 104-115°F).

Stir in commercial yoghurt or powdered acidophilus. Mix well. Pour into a wide mouthed vacuum flask and leave for eight hours or until thick. Once thickened, store in a refrigerator. Alternatively, pour into glass jars and surround with lukewarm water in an insulated bucket to keep at correct temperature for the culture to develop.

Remember to reserve 1 tablespoon of this yoghurt to use as the starter for the next batch. The next 3 or 4 batches can be made using your own starter culture. If the yoghurt starts to get too thin or the flavour deteriorates, start again with a new starter culture from the commercial yoghurt or the acidophilus powder.

Note: It is very important to sterilise all equipment when making milk cultures. A simple method is to rub with salt and then pour boiling water over the equipment.

Yoghurt Curd Cheese

Line a plastic sieve with muslin and place over a bowl to collect liquid. Pour yoghurt onto muslin and fold edges of cloth over to cover it. Leave it in refrigerator for about 8 hours or until the curd cheese is at the desired consistency.

Use as required.

Chopped herbs mixed through this cottage cheese makes a nice spread for unleavened bread. It has a firmer consistency than yoghurt so can be added to so many recipes, such as the basis for simple dips or salads. Ideal served with pasta, egg noodles or rice. See egg noodle recipe on page 32.

The whey liquid that has drained away can be used in soups or to boil rice or pasta for added nutrition.

Watermelon Yoghurt Smoothy

½ cup natural yoghurt
1 cup watermelon, roughly chopped, seed removed

Method: Place both ingredients into a bowl and blend to a smooth liquid. Chill well, if necessary, before serving. Yields 2 glasses. Substitute any fruit you desire. To sweeten if required, add several sultanas when blending.

Fromage Blanc

2 tablespoons cottage cheese or quark
2 tablespoons yoghurt or cold pressed flax oil
Squeeze lemon juice

Method: Place all ingredients into a blender and blend until smooth. Fromage Blanc is used extensively in France as a fat free substitute for cream to enrich sauces. It is also a way of taking uncooked oils so necessary in our food.

Make Your Own Cottage Cheese

Number 1 — guide method

1 cup Carnation skim milk powder
1 litre pure water
2 lemons, juiced

Method: Mix milk powder with water and heat in saucepan until lukewarm (40-46°C or 104-115°F). Add lemon juice and stand for 30 minutes until cool.

Line a strainer with a piece of muslin and strain the cheese. Refrigerate the cottage cheese and use as required. It is delicious mixed with fresh chopped chives, or fresh herbs or fruit such as pineapple or alternatively orange segments.

The whey can be used as stock or to cook rice in for extra flavour and nutrition. If you find the cottage cheese is a little too dry add some natural yoghurt.

Note: It is very important to sterilise all equipment when making milk cultures. A simple method is to rub with salt and then pour boiling water over the equipment. For the muslin used to strain the mixture simply boil in water to sterilise.

Make Your Own Cottage Cheese

Number 2 — enriched

1 cup Carnation skim milk powder
1 litre pure water
1 tablespoon sour cream
Juice ½ lemon

Method: Mix milk powder with water and heat in saucepan until lukewarm (40-46°C or 104-115°F). Stir in the sour cream and lemon juice.

Pour into a bowl and allow to stand at room temperature overnight, until the milk is set into a thick curd. Cut the curd several times right to the bottom of the dish.

Place the bowl in warm water for 1 hour or until curd feels just warm. Add more hot water, if necessary, as it cools down. Stir gently from time to time to keep temperature even. Line a strainer with a piece of muslin and strain the cheese. Allow to drain for at least an hour or until the cottage cheese has reached the desired consistency.

Place cottage cheese in a bowl and cover. Refrigerate until required. It will keep for about one week in the refrigerator.

Flavourings such as mixed fresh herbs, chives, shallots, capsicum or pineapple are delicious mixed into the cheese. If pineapple is not permitted on the program substitute another fruit of your choice such as orange segments.

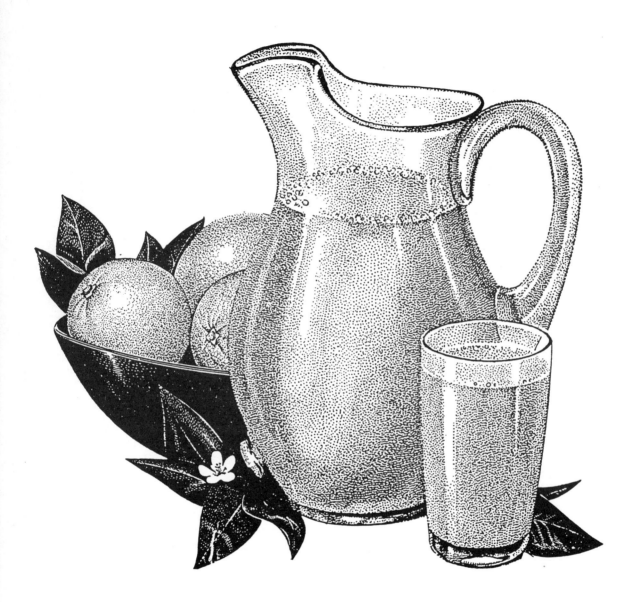

Fresh Juices

If making green juice always use one fruit juice with only one green at first to test compatibility. Add another green day by day, then if something disagrees you know which is the culprit. Experiment and keep a log of your favourites.

All ingredients should be washed carefully.

Juice together to make 250g (8oz), of any 2 or more of the following:

> Carrot, beetroot and tops, celery, parsley, spinach, one of the cabbage family, asparagus, lettuce, broccoli, choko, green beans, pineapple, grapes, apple.

The following are some nice combinations (plus apple or grape):

> Celery, broccoli.
> Choko, grapes.
> Lettuce, beetroot.
> Pineapple, spinach.
> Parsley, apple, green beans.
> Carrot, celery, lettuce.
> Celery, beetroot, carrot.
> Spinach, celery, lettuce.
> Cabbage, beetroot, choko.
> Capsicum, parsley, spinach.
> Cabbage, celery, carrot and apple.

Some Juice Favourites

1 part carrot, 1 part apple (green type).

3 parts carrot, 1 part celery.

3 parts carrot, 1 part cabbage (green).

1 part tomato, 1 part carrot.

2 parts cucumber, 1 part beetroot, 1 part apple.

2 parts grape, 1 part choko, 1 cucumber or zucchini.

All watermelon, with rind too.

1 part carrot, 2 parts apple, 1 to 2 whole limes.

3 parts orange, $\frac{1}{2}$ part apple lettuce green, $\frac{1}{2}$ part broccoli.

2 parts pineapple, $1\frac{1}{2}$ parts cabbage, $\frac{1}{2}$ part comfrey.

2 parts pear, 1 part cabbage, 1 part choko or zucchini.

2 parts apple, 1 part guava, 1 part zucchini.

2 parts apple, 1 part pear, 1 part guava.

2 parts grape, 2 parts choko.

2 parts carrot, 2 parts beetroot.

1 part celery, 1 part beans, 1 part zucchini, 1 part apple.

1 part cucumber, 1 part capsicum, 1 part silverbeet, 1 part apple.

2 parts apple, 1 part celery, 1 part beetroot.

1 part grape, 1 part celery, 1 part choko, 1 part apple.

2 parts grape, 1 part carrot, 1 part apple.

Herb Teas

Use any of the following:

Lemon balm, chamomile, peppermint, valerian, red clover, lemon grass and chaperal, samshu and fresh herbs such as basil, sage, thyme and rosemary may be used as any combination that suits your palate.

Commercial teas made from barley and chickory are suitable as a hot drink but not as a substitute for raw fresh and vegetable juices.

Liver Juice

As a boost to the immune system, liver is unequalled.

The liver is the kitchen of the body, home of many different sorts of cells all with varied tasks to perform. Among the many hundreds of transactions it monitors is the making and the breaking down of our sex hormones out of the raw product, cholesterol. It also detoxifies substances harmful to the body and excretes the products of detoxification into the bile to be passed out into the intestine for elimination. An even more important job that the liver performs is the manufacture of "tumor necrosis factor" and other enzymes that allow the immune system to function in its task of destroying damaging substances in the body, cancer cells for instance.

The macrophages and other white cells that are made and contained in the liver are still alive in fresh raw liver. The anti-blocking agent or tumor necrosis factor, is still present if the liver has not been frozen and is a major deterrent to the spread of cancer.

The aim in taking raw liver juice is to gain these substances for those with cancer who are not making sufficient for their own body's needs.

Calves liver is used because it is not as strong tasting as lambs fry, and makes a thinner and more palatable juice. In fact, fresh young unfrozen liver when juiced with carrot, tastes of carrot. It may also be juiced with apple for those who find carrot unpalatable. Also young animals have not been subjected to toxic substances and have not contracted diseases.

Dr Max Gerson who found liver juice so important for his patients in the first half of the century, believed that the only way of making liver juice was to use the grind and press type of machine, such as the Norwalk juicer, which did not heat the substances going through it or alter their electrical potential. In his day, the slow and clumsy centrifugal juicers tended to do this.

However, the grind and press juicers are now far too expensive for most people to buy and the centrifugal ones are not only cheap but also have a less destructive effect on the substances being juiced than they used to have. People are getting better using either nowadays, but the liver juice must be drunk almost immediately it is made or it will oxidise and destroy some of the important items in it.

Those who do not like the taste may take liver juice without tasting it by using the following methods:

1. Make and stand aside a small amount of carrot, apple or grape juice before starting with the liver. Hold the nose and drink the liver and carrot juice down promptly. Then before releasing the nose clear the palate by drinking the apple chaser. Then take another breath.
2. Alternatively, just drink the juice down then take the chaser without taking a breath if lung capacity is large enough to do that.

It helps to know that the substances extracted from fresh liver cost $680 a day to have by injection if you could get them.

That makes it taste much better!

If the thought of raw liver is so abhorrent that it makes you feel nauseous then forget it! You probably would not digest it properly if you did take it.

However the benefit of taking raw liver juice with carrot is the tremendous boost it gives to the immune system. For this effect the liver must be from a very young calf, unfrozen and taken as raw juice within three days of slaughter only. Check the source of supply very carefully.

If liver is not available at all take a freeze dried liver tablet daily. It is not as good of course but it is better than no liver at all.

Liver and Carrot Juice

$\frac{1}{2}$ peeled apple or $\frac{1}{2}$ lemon, sliced
50 to 250g raw unfrozen young calf liver
3 to 6 carrots washed

Method: Start with 50g of liver — you won't even taste it. Cut liver into thin strips, cut carrot long ways into thin strips. Put each strip of liver through the juicer with two strips of carrot. Strain the juice through a fine sieve. Drink immediately. Clear the palate with either apple or slices of lemon.

Warning: It is most unwise to use lambs liver since sheep in Australia are subject to liver fluke in some areas. Calves do not harbour liver fluke.

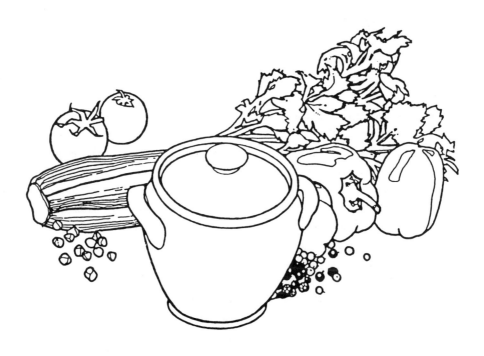

Garlic and Onion

Garlic and Onion have long been used medicinally, predating written history.

Grown in the right soil both will contain the *essential trace elements, selenium* and *germanium,* with their healing anti-oxidant powers. Both also contain a healing substance, allicin, which is manufactured in them by the combination of enzymes allinase and allicin. It is allicin that has the strong odour.

Onions have about one-tenth the amount of allicin that is in garlic, so by volume onions are used in larger amounts.

For culinary purposes these substances can be most effective when eaten raw in salads, dressings, mayonnaise and sauces. They may also be cooked in any savoury dish to give flavour and nutriment.

However, it is wise to eat garlic always with other food since too much allicin can be irritating to some stomachs on its own.

Historically, the Codes Ebers, an Egyptian papyrus of about 1550 B.C., includes 22 remedies containing garlic as an effective formula for a variety of ailments such as heart problems, headache, worms, tumors and bites.

Ancient Greeks Aristotle, Hippocrates and Aristophanes all discussed the therapeutic effects of garlic and onions. Dioscorides, the Roman physician of First Century A.D., prescribed it as a treatment for intestinal worms for the Roman soldiers.

It was (and still is) used by athletes as a motivator and stimulant. Antiseptic garlic lotions are used in India for cleansing wounds and ulcers. Onion tea is recommended in China for fever, headache, cholera and dysentry. Louis Pasteur confirmed the antibacterial activity of garlic and Albert Schweitzer used it against dysentry in his African hospital.

It is still widely used for its anti-fungal properties for some forms of vaginitis and dermatitis.

The anti-thromboic factor in onions as well as garlic have been used throughout history to treat and prevent blood clots. Numerous studies in India, United States, Russia, China and elsewhere have now proved the efficacy of many of the folk remedies.

Even so, there are those who love and those who hate the onion family. To be most effective, garlic should be eaten raw. The sulphur containing molecules of the amino acid 1 cysteine which is the precursor for the odoriferous and tear-producing substrates that form after cutting or crushing, are excreted through the breath and the perspiration if taken in large quantities. Some people find these properties so unpleasant that they outweigh the therapeutic uses.

Cooking can change some molecules and reduce this unpleasant quality. Taking chlorophyll in the form of pungent herbs such as parsley, mint and thyme can also inhibit the strong odour somewhat. A little may be appetising, whereas too much may be repugnant.

Note: "Recipe for Salad" written by Sydney Smith, the 19th century essayist:

> *"Let onions atoms lurk within the bowl*
> *and scarce suspected animate the whole."*

Wheatgrass

Wheatgrass contains the highest amount of abscisic acid — a substance that inhibits the growth hormone that cancer cells make. It is a good substance to juice for this reason. There are many other easily digestible nutrients dissolved in wheatgrass juice too, but abscisic acid (dormin) is the most important. There are useful amounts of beta-carotene, chlorophyl, vitamins B_1, B_2, B_3, C and E with some calcium phosphorous, nitrogen, flavins and other substances not yet identified.

To grow it:

Take a cardboard or styrene foam avocado or mango tray, or cut down a tall box to 3.5″ deep and put in it a liner of plastic and 1″ of garden soil, sand with 50% compost added of potting mixture.

Wash well, seed wheat from the produce agent to remove fungicides or chemicals. Soak the wheat well covered with water for about 12 hours. Moisten soil with water. Spread wheat thickly on the dirt, cover with sheets of damp newspaper. Cover with a plastic sheet to keep the moisture in.

After a few days the wheat has sprouted.

Remove the covers and water daily.

Allow to grow in indirect sunlight.

It is ready to cut for juicing when 4″ to 7″ high, before two stalks form.

Cut with scissors at a point about 1″ above the dirt or where green begins.

A 2″ strip of cut wheatgrass should make about 2 oz of juice.

Do not drink more than this at first. You may work up slowly to 8 oz of juice daily if this has been advised on your program.

If using a special juicer like a mincer, worked by hand or by electricity, the directions are with the machine.

If using a centrifugal juicer, care must be taken not to clog the machine and burn out the motor.

Experiment with these ways of extracting juice:

1. Bruise the cut grass, rolling it into tight ¼″ bundles in the hands before feeding it into the juicer, little by little. Do not overload the machine.

2. Cut the grass into 1″ pieces, roll up bundles of cut grass in lettuce leaves before feeding them into the machine. Drink immediately.

3. Cut wheatgrass into ½″ lengths. Dice ½″ peeled apple. Put batches of wheatgrass into blender with apple and about 1″ or more of pure water. Make a pureé. Take a clean piece of sheeting about 1 foot square, lie it across the top of jug and push down to make a depression in the centre.

   Pour the pureé into the cloth gently, little by little, to strain the juice holding the edges to stop them falling into the jug. When mostly strained, take up the edges of the cloth and wring the rest of the fluid out into the jug.

   Drink immediately to prevent oxidation. It tastes good with the apple in it.

Wheatgrass juice is so easily absorbed it is best to take it alone about one hour before, or two hours after eating to gain the best from it. It may be mixed with other raw juice to alter the taste.

It should never be cooked. It loses a proportion of its nutrients if kept, even in the refrigerator, after preparation.

Food Guidelines For Those With Cancer

	Foods to Include	*Foods to Avoid*
Beverages	Large amounts of all fresh vegetable and fruit juices, especially carrot, greens, beet and apple. Herb teas, especially peppermint.	All canned, frozen and artficial fruit drinks. Alcohol, cocoa, tea and coffee.
Breads	Millet, rye, buckwheat, wholemeal wheat, corn, lupin and soya. Corn tortillas. Only 100% grains, freshly ground or sprouted, free of additives. Avoid rancid flour. Use a flour mill.	White bread and white flour products such as macaroni, crackers and snack food.
Cereals	Millet, oatmeal, rye, brown rice, barley, buckwheat, corn, wheat. Avoid rancid grains. Use a nut grinder or flour mill.	Processed cereals, which are ready cooked or flaked, puffed, etc. White rice.
Dairy	Unsweetened yoghurt, kefir, certified cream, cottage cheese, freeze dried skim milk or raw, unhomogenised certified milk. Butter mixed with cold pressed oil.	Salty, fatty cheeses and commercial milk.
Eggs	Free-range eggs, poached, boiled (with yolk runny) scrambled, cooked on low heat or custards.	All "battery" and fried eggs.
Fruits	All fresh fruits (organically grown): apples, apricots, bananas, cherries berries, melon, papaya, pineapple, etc., etc. Wash well or peel.	Sprayed, sweetened, glace, frozen and canned fruit. Sulphured dried fruits unless washed.
Flesh Protein	Fresh fish, rabbit, turkey (naturally raised). Grilled, broiled or baked; fresh lambs or calf liver and kidney.	Shellfish and all other meats. Fried, smoked, salted or processed meats. No nitrates antibiotic or stilbesterol.
Oils	Most cold-pressed unsaturated oils such as linseed (flax), safflower, sesame, corn, soya, olive and avocado. Used sparingly. Avocado used whole may replace butter.	Cotton seed oil. Rancid refined or heating oil. Shortening or margarine. Fried Foods.
Nuts	Most fresh raw nuts, particularly, almonds, macadamias, walnuts and pecans. Raw nut butters freshly made refrigerated to avoid rancidity. Use sparingly.	Roasted and salted nuts, especially peanuts. Rancid nut and nut butters.

	Foods to Include	*Foods to Avoid*
Seasonings	Herbs; chives, garlic, parsley, bay, basil, sage, thyme, savoury. Kelp and vegetable seasonings.	Salt. Commercially prepared sauces, etc. with preservative, MSG, sodium nitrate and metabisulphate.
Seeds	Sunflower, pumpkin, sesame, pine and flax. Fruit kernels, apricot, apple, prune, plum and peach, etc.	Roasted and salted seeds.
Sprouts & Legumes	Mung, sunflower, lentil, soy beans, fenugreek, buckwheat and wheat, which can be made into wheatgrass juice. All edible bean and pea family.	Potato sprouts
Sweets	Malted sorghum, rice, raw honey, pure maple syrup, date sugar and carob used sparingly over cereal or in desserts (with healthy ingredients)	White sugar and sugar containing foods and substitutes. Commercial candies and pastries.
Vegetables	All raw or cooked vegetables. Homemade soups. Salads, use lavishly.	Sprayed, frozen and canned vegetables. Fried potato and corn chips, containing cooked fats and preservatives.
Water	Pure water, purified spring or rain or distilled water or purified by osmosis or sunlight. Boiling destroys some common germs and toxins.	Tap water, even boiled.

This diet can be more or less restricted according to the severity of the disease. Eliminate all animal products, e.g. dairy and meat during the first 3 weeks of detoxification. Read "Heal Cancer" also by Ruth Cilento for more information.

"Heal Cancer: Choose Your Own Survival Path".

Dr. Ruth Cilento, P.O. Box 129 Bracken Ridge, Queensland 4017.

Published by Hill of Content, 86 Bourke Street, Melbourne, 3000.